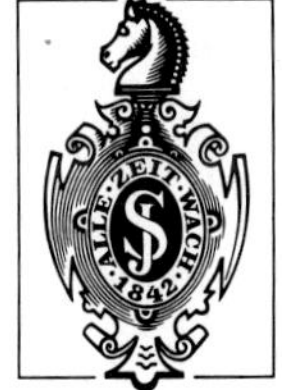

B. von Barsewisch

Perinatal Retinal Haemorrhages

Morphology, Aetiology and Significance

Foreword by O.-E. Lund

With 64 Figures and 13 Plates

Springer-Verlag
Berlin Heidelberg New York 1979

Professor Dr. med. BERNHARD VON BARSEWISCH
a-pl. Professor der Ludwig-Maximilians-Universität München,
Chefarzt der Augenklinik Herzog Carl Theodor,
8000 München 2

ISBN 3-540-09167-X Springer-Verlag Berlin Heidelberg New York
ISBN 0-387-09167-X Springer-Verlag New York Heidelberg Berlin

Library of Congress Cataloging in Publication Data: Barsewisch, Bernhard von, 1935–
Perinatal retinal haemorrhages. First version written in German as Habilitationsschrift,
Munich. Bibliography: p. Includes index. 1. Pediatric opthalmology. 2. Retina—Hemor-
rhage. 3. Infants (Newborn)—Diseases. I. Title. [DNLM: 1. Infant, Newborn, Diseases. 2.
Retinal hemorrhage—In infancy and childhood. WW270 B282p] RE48.2.C5B37
618.9′209′73 78-25767

Offsetprinting and Binding: Konrad Triltsch, Würzburg
2123/3130-543210

*To my teachers
Professor Dr. G. Meyer-Schwickerath
Professor Dr. O.-E. Lund*

Foreword

Retinal haemorrhage occurring during birth is a common feature in the newborn. There is no basic funduscopic or morphologic difference between this perinatal type of haemorrhage and that in the adult. The difference is that perinatal haemorrhage resorbs rapidly, within a few days, and no functional defects of retinal vessels are known.

The first observation of perinatal haemorrhage took place nearly 100 years ago. Many observations have been published in short papers; what was still lacking was a systematic pathogenic classification of the different types of haemorrhage, a comparison of the perinatal type of other types of retinal haemorrhage, a comparison to other perinatal ocular haemorrhages, a detailed histologic description and a multi-faceted correlation of haemorrhage to aetiologic factors.

The author has based his comprehensive evaluation on the observation of more than 400 newborn infants, the reexamination of several cases with macular haemorrhage, the histologic work-up of serial sections and the review of extensive literature.

It is a remarkable fact that a physiologic process, birth, is related to this type of vessel rupture, which is present during a short period of postnatal life. In its complex analysis of these facts and conditions this book is particularly valuable.

Munich, Winter 1978/79   O.-E. LUND

Acknowledgements

I would like to express my sincere thanks to those who supported me in collecting literature: Dr. I. Wallow (Madison/USA); Dr. T. Takahashi (Kobe/Japan); Dr. G. Theodossiades (Athens/Greece); Dr. A. Alexandridis (Munich); Frau Dr. B. Kuschel (Munich); the Institut Chibret (Clermont-Ferrand/France) and the "Internationale Schritfttumsbeschaffung Kröhnke-Heyer" (Heidelberg).

While able to read the Romance languages himself, the author is greatly indebted to all those who have helped by translating languages unknown to him:

Japanese: Dr. Takahashi (Kobe)
Russian: Frau Dr. K. Kernt, Frau Dr. E. Haritoglou and Dr. R. Adamczyk (Munich)
Polish: Frau Dozentin Selman (Munich)
Czech: Frau Dr. Simon (Munich)
Slovak: Frau A. Lauova (Munich)
Hungarian: Dr. F. Lajosi, Dr. I. Richter (Munich)
Greek: Dr. A. Souvatzoglou (Athens), Dr. A. Alexandridis (Munich)
Hebrew: Frau K. Wasserstein (Munich)

The first version of this monograph was written in German as a "Habilitationsschrift" (a paper, part of which fulfilled the requirement for becoming "Privatdozent" of the University of Munich). I would like to express my gratitute to Professor Dr. O.-E. Lund, who helped me a great deal by his cooperative counselling in my first attempt to order the vast amount of material. For correcting my English manuscript I am greatly indebted to cand med. R. Simon.

My thanks have to be extended too to the colleagues who helped me in taking fundus photographs (Dr. U. Schum, Dr. J.-H. Greite, Dr. V.P. Gabel), to Dr. Stefani for help in pathoanatomic work and to Dr. I. Wallow for his aid in electron-microscopic preparations. I would also like to express my thanks for the cooperation of the histology laboratory and the photographic department of our hospital, and last but certainly not least to thank Frau I. Mannl, who with patience and accuracy typed the first and the second versions of the German and now the English text.

Contents

Introduction

The perinatal period is a particularly dangerous one. Its scientific investigation and the medical care of mother and child have been intensified in recent years and denominated "perinatal medicine". The most important research in this branch of medical science has been contributed by obstetricians and paediatricians, but relations to other fields are also very close as, for example, in the neurologic and haematologic abnormalities of the newborn.

Opththalmology can also contribute to perinatal medicine not only by observing the nerve-head and the retinal vessels, which link ophthalmology to so many other medical branches, but also by revealing a most spectacular abnormality which occurs in a high percentage of newborn infants: perinatal retinal haemorrhages. These can be so extensive that the posterior half of the retina shows more haemorrhagic areas than normal ones. If not related to birth, a similar ophthalmoscopic appearance would correspond to a severe disease such as subarachnoid haemorrhage or central venous occlusion. But here the newborn infants affected are otherwise healthy and the haemorrhages absorb rapidly.

This type of retinal effusion was first described in 1881 and since then its morphology, aetiology and significance have been under discussion. The literature contains the most divergent opinions and speculations on these three topics. This study has been carried out to provide more facts and thereby give the discussion a more substantival basis.

Clear results were to be expected from a thorough morphologic analysis. Clinical observations of many disorders of the newborn had not led to a valid morphologic classification. Fundus photography proved to be superior, and with continuous serial sections correlated with the photographs a great number of new details were revealed.

Evaluating the importance of aetiologic factors is far more difficult. Here, many suspected correlations were a result of having examined too few cases, e.g. the simple question of whether more boys or more girls were affected found contradictory answers.

Practically no two clinical series correspond to each other. A review of the world literature was attempted, including the most remote publications available. This extensive compilation finally revealed indications as to which factors really influence the incidence of retinal haemorrhages.

A correlation of retinal and intracranial haemorrhages in the newborn would have been of the greatest significance; but the original results have not been confirmed by later authors. Another suspected correlation of macular haemorrhages and later amblyopia has been discussed by many, but only investigated by a few authors. The reliable data published about the course of macular haemorrhages are disappointing. Besides that, discussions on sequelae were based more on speculations than on pathoanatomic details. The most valuable histologic examination of this type of haemorrhages dates from 1890 (Naumoff).

So what began as a very limited investigation on the influence of fibrinolysis inhibitors on perinatal retinal haemorrhages developed further and further, especially when with reading more literature the number of contradictions grew and the amount of clarifications did not. The author felt a monograph on this subject would be useful and of interest not only to ophthalmologists but also to paediatricians and obstetricians and all those concerned with perinatal problems. It should be stressed that this book is not composed of material from previous papers but that most of the information is being published for the first time. The author, a specialist in ophthalmology, apologizes for less competent handling of themes less familiar to him (e.g. obstetrics or haematology).

Perinatal retinal haemorrhages have the advantages that they can be easily observed and that their study is not bound to large hospital centres. The disadvantage is that some publications are of a very low scientific standard and that other good papers are difficult to obtain. Unfortunately some authors owe their frequent quotation more to the easy accessibility of their paper than to its importance, whereas other very thorough studies remain practically unknown.

I. The First Observation

A. Königstein or von Jaeger?

The first author to describe retinal haemorrhages in newborn infants was L. Königstein in the year 1881. All later investigators up to the 1920s gave Königstein the credit for the first description. Since then opinion is split into two different groups. Only a few continue to cite Königstein — which is correct — (Powelett and Townes, 1948; Candian, 1949; Grassi and Musini, 1950; Yoshioka, 1954; Schwartz, 1961; Yohidta et al., 1961; Veinbaum, 1967; Wierhake, 1971).

Most of the other authors (e.g. Lachmann, 1927 quoting Jacobs, 1924; Edgerton, 1934; Jarny, 1947; Dolcet-Buxeres and Ferrer-Pi, 1954; Crehange, 1958; Brogi et al., 1962; Grigera, 1964; Kobayashi et al., 1964; Jain and Gupta, 1965; Pannarale, 1966; Schenker and Gombos, 1966; Stefanini et al., 1968; Takeda, 1968; Sezen, 1970; Schlaeder et al., 1971; Bergen and Margolis, 1976) believe that von Jaeger gave the first description in 1861. Unfortunately Duke-Elder also repeats this error in his *System of Ophthalmology* (1967).

What could be the source of this confusion? The original publications, i.e. von Jaeger's book *Die Einstellung des dioptrischen Apparates im menschlichen Auge* [1] (1861) and Königstein's article *Untersuchungen an den Augen neugeborener Kinder* [2] (1881), are not easily accessible. Therefore the error must be due to continuous repetitions of a wrong quotation. Investigation leads to Eherenfest's very influential book, *Birth Injuries of the Child* (1922). Ehrenfest mentioned in the context of perinatal retinal haemorrhages von Jaeger's work of 1861. But the connection is different. Ehrenfest said only that von Jaeger examined newborn babies, but not that he noted retinal haemorrhages, as subsequent authors believed. Also Könistein's paper is mentioned by Ehrenfest in a different context, and it seems that Ehrenfest had seen neither of the original publications.

It is debatable whether von Jaeger saw the haemorrhages. His book, which is not easy to read, deals with the refraction of the human eye. To compare different age groups he also examined 50 children aged 9—16 days in a foundling hospital. With this late examination date, only relics of very massive fundus haemorrhages could have been found. In addition his technique with a direct ophthalmoscope and without mydriatics was not appropriate to reveal haemorrhages. Both this technique and his refractive results were severly attacked by later authors (Ely, 1880; Königstein, 1881; Schleich, 1894; von Sicherer, 1907). Furthermore, in his atlas *Ergebnisse der Untersuchung mit dem Augenspiegel* [3] (1876), von Jaeger did not mention the haemorrhages in

---

1   The adaptation of the dioptric apparatus of the human eye.
2   Investigation of the eyes of newborns.
3   Results of Ophthalmoscopy.

question. But without any doubt Duke-Elder's citation "Retinal haemorrhages in the newborn, as first recorded and illustrated by von Jaeger (1861) . . . " will continue to cause confusion.

On the other hand Königstein clearly claims to give the first report on retinal haemorrhages in newborn infants. The main purpose of his presentation, as he gave it at a conference in Vienna (according to Schleich in May 1881), was the discussion of von Jager's questionable refractive results. Königstein applied atropine and his results are in accordance with the general opinion about the refraction in the eye of newborn children. Because of its difficult accessibility, the translated text of the first description of retinal haemorrhages follows (c.f. original German text in the Appendix):

Very frequently one encounters indistinct red patches of different size and shape. In the beginning I could not explain these. Owing to the difficulty in observing one area over a longer time, I was uncertain whether I was dealing with extravasations or whether the pigment epithelium was defective in one place. I reexamined several of these cases after a few days but could no longer find any trace of the patches. In one infant that I examined a few hours after birth, I found two dark red patches, whose size was nearly that of a disc diameter, close to the optic disc. I could identify these as extravasations of blood. I reexamined the infant each day, observing how the extravasations from the periphery as well as the centre grew lighter, thus becoming indistinct. I observed this in several children. In children a few days old, the patches were more or less dark red, distinctly outlined, frequently protruding into the vitreous body, whereas slightly older children demonstrated only indistinct patches. Extravasations of blood are not rare; I have observed them in 10% of my cases and am surprised that they have escaped the observation of other investigators. Either they are found in radial orientation, forming streaks that accompany vessels, or in small or larger patches of circular configuration. Frequently the entire fundus is covered. As mentioned above, they are rapidly reabsorbed and are therefore of no further significance. Nevertheless, it could be possible that, with extensive extravasation, retinal elements are destroyed and that the extravasations could be the cause of later amblyopia without other findings. When do the extravasations occur and how are they produced? They certainly do not begin during uterine life. Their appearance and analogy with effusions into skin and conjunctiva make this unlikely. They can only occur during birth or as a result of the blood circulation's being altered by the first breaths. The great pressure exerted on the infant makes the occurrence of haemorrhage likely during birth. It must be mentioned, however, that in difficult forceps deliveries, in frontal presentations and with large heavy children, haemorrhages are no more frequently observed than with small or immature children, delivered relatively easily and quickly. It is my opinion that the cause of haemorrhage is the change in circulation and the arteriolization of blood. Frequently enough I had the opportunity to observe how, in a child who was blue (venous) at birth and turned pink after a few breaths, numerous extravasations developed in the skin. The same process is likely to happen in the retina.

Thus Königstein not only gives a description of the appearance, but already discusses later amblyopia and gives a first theory about the origin of these haemorrhages, namely via arteriolization of the blood.

In 1884 Schleich was the next author to mention these haemorrhages, saying that little could be added to the statements of Königstein, who saw them first. As mentioned before, several authors who knew Königstein's text in the original mention his first description (Coburn, 1904; Leber, 1915).

B. Ely

Reviewing more contemporary literature the writer found an article by the American ophthalmologist E.T. Ely, which seems to indicate that in reality he was the first to see, though not clearly to describe, a perinatal retinal haemorrhage. His "Ophthalmoscopic observations upon the refraction of the eyes of newly-born children" was published in the *Archives of Ophthalmology,* 1880. Most of the children in his study were too old to demonstrate haemorrhages. Of the nine he saw within the first 24 h of life, one, in the author's opinion, clearly had perinatal retinal haemorrhages. These were still persistent at the second day and had dissolved within 3 weeks. Ely's original text reads:

In case No. 63 there was marked neuro-retinitis in the right eye. The history of this case was as follows: The child was left upon the steps of the Foundling Asylum one cold night in January. Having been left at the wrong door, it was not discovered until two o'clock in the morning. It was then so chilled that it was revived only with difficulty. It had not been washed and was evidently only a few hours old. It was seen by me in the afternoon of the same day. It was a small baby, of "senile" appearance; otherwise, the general examination showed nothing abnormal. The ophthalmoscope revealed marked evidences of neuro-retinitis in the right eye. The optic disc and surrounding retina were much swollen; the retinal veins enlarged and tortuous. Scattered over the fundus were some small hemorrhages, and a few round, yellowish spots, looking like exsudations. There was slight divergence of the optic axes.

This confusing case history, and the exceptional diagnosis, which was never again to be established in the thousands of other children examined, make it understandable that later authors like Königstein (1881) and von Sicherer (1907) were convinced that Ely had seen none of these haemorrhages.

C. Summary

Contrary to the general opinion, based on repeated wrong quotations, von Jaeger (1961) did not see or describe retinal haemorrhages in newborn children. The American ophthalmologist Ely (1880) seems to have seen a case but published it with the confusing diagnosis of neuro-retinitis. The first clear description of the perinatal retinal haemorrhages dated from 1881 and was given by Königstein.

Zusammenfassung

Entgegen der allgemeinen Ansicht, die nur auf Wiederholungen falscher Zitate beruht,
hat von Jaeger (1861) Netzhautblutungen bei Neugeborenen nicht gesehen und nicht
beschrieben. Der amerikanische Ophthalmologe Ely scheint 1880 einen Fall gesehen zu
haben, wurde jedoch wegen der verwirrenden Diagnose Neuro-Retinitis nicht als Erst-
beschreiber angesehen. Die erste klare Beschreibung der perinatalen Netzhautblutungen
wurde 1881 von Königstein gegeben.

II. Material and Methods

A. Ophthalmoscopy

Four hundred newborn infants of the I. Frauenklinik der Universität München were examined within the first 24 h of life. A first series of 265 children was seen in 1969, consisting of mature infants after spontaneous delivery from occipital presentation. The purpose was to compare a group without treatment to a group of children whose mothers received an injection of a fibrinolysis inhibitor before the onset of labour. Rationale and results of this method will be discussed in the section on haemorrhagic diathesis (Chap. VII, D, Sect. 4). According to a review of more literature at that time, opinions about perinatal retinal haemorrhages were most controversial. For an independent evaluation a new series seemed desirable, comparing different types of delivery. The final number of children seen was 400. Of these, 200 served as the normal control group, and form the basis for discussing the obstetric, maternal and infantile factors influencing the incidence of retinal haemorrhages.

Ophthalmoscopy was carried out with a strong monocular ophthalmoscope (Bonnoskop, F. Eischeid/Bonn), using an aspheric lens of 16 D. With this method, centre and mid-periphery of the fundus were easily accessible, and the temporal and nasal equatorial periphery could be visualized. This indirect ophthalmoscopy with brillant contrast keeps the retina in view despite constant eye movements, frequently encountered in the newborn. All infants were examined within the first 24 h of life. Some of them were reexamined after several days to confirm the well-known rapid dissolution of these haemorrhages. Ophthalmoscopy was carried out with fully dilated pupils. Although one drop of a mydriatic well applied is sufficient, the nurses were asked to apply two different agents at an interval of 10 min [Mydriaticum (Roche) and Neosynephrine (Winthrop)]. This method was used to make sure that at least one application was effective and proved to be very successful. To immobilize the arms, the child was wrapped in a blanket ("mummified"). The nurse would then position the head with both hands, holding the two small specula (Desmarres), which had been inserted by the ophthalmologist.

The ophthalmoscopic observations were noted, together with the clinical data of mother and child and the course of delivery. Distribution, number of special aspects of haemorrhages were noted. Up to 20 haemorrhages were counted, and higher numbers were estimated. Macular affection was meticulously noted, since so many other reports are inexact on this point.

B. Fundus Photography

The fundus of selected children was photographed, especially when the macula was involved. For this purpose the children were brought with dilated pupils to the University Eye Hospital (Augenklinik der Universität). The children were placed in a supine position under a hanging Zeiss fundus camera, which is used for fluorescein angiography (Remky and Schum, 1968). Eccentric fundus areas were visualized by tilting the head and guiding the eye with a squint hook (Bulpitt and Baum, 1969). Besides the text illustrations, the composite photographs thus obtained appear as Plates I–IX in the Appendix (see page 144 ff).

Besides colour photographs, primary black and white negatives demonstrated the haemorrhages very clearly. Remaining technical defects are due to the incomplete immobilization of the children's eyes. These photographs, obtained with a hanging fundus camera, seem to be superior to those obtained with a hand-held camera (cf. the illustrations by Kobayashi et al., 1964; Krebs and Jaeger, 1966; Takeda, 1968; Tranou-Sphalangakou, 1968; Wierhake, 1971). Bulpitt and Baum (1969) changed from a hand camera to a Zeiss camera. The fundus photographs proved to be extremely helpful in interpreting histologic and ophthalmoscopic findings, i.e. with the knowledge of the details from the photographs clinical judgement was more precise and valuable. Since photography is so much superior to ophthalmoscopy, it goes without saying that fundus paintings as first presented by von Sicherer (1907) cannot have the same value.

C. Histology

The eyes of eight children who died within a few hours to 3 days after birth were examined histologically. In four of these no haemorrhage was visible. The other four had retinal haemorrhages in both eyes. Two of these were immature infants and their retinae showed marked autolytic alterations. These latter were only used as a means of comparison. The illustrations of the post mortem retinae and the histologic specimen were taken from two children whose eyes had been enucleated shortly after death.

The strongest similarity with the clinically observed more extensive haemorrhages was found in a child with a birth weight of 1810 g and a length of 42 cm. It had died half an hour after forceps delivery due to other complications. The overall appearance of the fundi is shwon in Plates X and XI.

The eyes were dissected either immediately after enucleation or after they had been partially fixed and then fundus photographs were taken. Some specimens were fixed in formaldehyde, others in glutaraldehyde. Specimens from both groups were embedded in paraffin. Material fixed in glutaraldehyde was also embedded in epon and 1-μm sections were cut with the LKB-microtome. These were stained with toluidine blue. Some originally formalin-fixed and paraffin-embedded specimens were reembedded in epon after postfixation in osmium tetroxide.

Ten-micron-thick serial sections of the paraffin-embedded material were prepared. This was necessary to reveal the vessel rupture within the sometimes rather extensive haemorrhages. The serial sections were stained with haematoxyline-eosine or Goldner.

PAS-stained slides were used to demonstrate the hyaloid membrane and intra-vascular fibrin coagula. The latter were also stained with PTAH (phospho-tungstic-acid-haematoxylin).

D. Clinical Follow-Up

Thirty-one children with clinically observed haemorrhages involving the macular area were reexamined at the age of 6 or 7 years. At this age cooperation was good, so that reliable results regarding visual acuity, binocular function and refractive errors were obtained. Fundus photographs of the central area were taken and compared with the topographic notes, drawings or fundus photographs taken within 24 h after birth. Visual acuity was tested at a Möller-Wedel clinical examination unit (Idem-Combi) with the Möller-Wedel phoropter and projector. Binocular functions were tested with the Titmus test and occasional additional examinations. To check whether amblyopia was caused by a refractive error; refractometry was performed with the Hartinger refractometer ("aus Jena"/GDR).

E. Summary

Four hundred newborn infants were examined within the first 24 h of life with indirect ophthalmoscopy and after pupil dilatation. Of these, 200 were delivered normally from occipital presentation. They form the control group, to be compared to other types of delivery and to a group in which a fibrinolysis inhibitor had been applied. Number and localization of retinal haemorrhages were thoroughly noted. In some cases of special interest fundus photographs were taken with a hanging Zeiss fundus camera. These in vivo photographs were compared to post mortem ones, which then were examined in serial sections. Thirty-one children with macular haemorrhages were reexamined at the age of 6 or 7 years.

Zusammenfassung

400 Neugeborene wurden innerhalb der ersten 24 Stunden unter Pupillenerweiterung mit indirekter Ophthalmoskopie untersucht. 200, die ohne Komplikationen aus Hinterhauptslage geboren wurden, bilden die Kontrollgruppe, die mit anderen Geburtsverläufen und einer Serie nach Anwendung eines Fibrinolyse-Inhibitors verglichen werden. Bei einigen besonders interessanten Fällen wurden Fundusfotografien mit einer hängend montierten Zeiss-Fundus-Kamera aufgenommen. Diese in vivo-Fotografien wurden mit post mortem-Fotografien der Netzhaut verglichen, die in Serienschnitten weiter untersucht wurden. 31 Kinder mit Blutungen der Macularegion wurden im Alter von 6 oder 7 Jahren nachuntersucht.

III. Morphology

Several authors tried to classify the retinal haemorrhages they found in newborn infants according to their different appearances. Most investigators differentiate two or more flat types of haemorrhage and one three-dimensional prominent type of effusion, normally denominated as "preretinal". Some of the features, like the flame-shaped appearance of haemorrhages in the nerve fibre layer, have been correctly described by many authors. For the rest, the descriptions remain incomplete or incorrect, varying from author to author, and their explanations are based on speculations.

Histologic documentation was not used to understand the clinical morphology of these haemorrhages, and the ophthalmoscopic appearance was not discussed in the histoplathologic investigations. A great step towards a better morphologic understanding of these perinatal retinal haemorrhages is offered by fundus photography. This reveals many details which can be clearly correlated with histopathologic pictures. Therefore the following morphologic classification is based on fundus photographs which are compared to post mortem retinae and documented by serial sections of these. In brief, there are three types of intraretinal haemorrhages and three types of extraretinal haemorrhages:

A. Intraretinal haemorrhages
    1. Flame-shaped haemorrhages of the nerve fibre layer
    2. Granular haemorrhages of the internal granular layer
    3. Hemispheric submembranacious haemorrhages
B. Extraretinal haemorrhages
    1. Subretinal haemorrhages
    2. Subhyaloid haemorrhages between internal limiting membrane and hyaloid membrane
    3. Hyaloid (vitreous) haemorrhages

A. Intraretinal Haemorrhages

The majority of perinatal retinal haemorrhages consist of intraretinal layers of blood cells. The effusion can originate from a rupture of a capillary in the internal granular layer or of a venule or capillary of the nerve fibre layer. Bleeding of these two layers practically always occurs simultaneously. Because of this and existing similarities, the ophthalmoscopic appearance of both types will be described together before discussing their histologic differences. Figures 1 and 2 illustrate the fresh state of these perinatal haemorrhages, as they were taken a few hours after birth.

Figure 1 shows the varying appearance and extent of the extravasations. In spite of all differences, the style of the configuration makes it possible to distinguish two types:

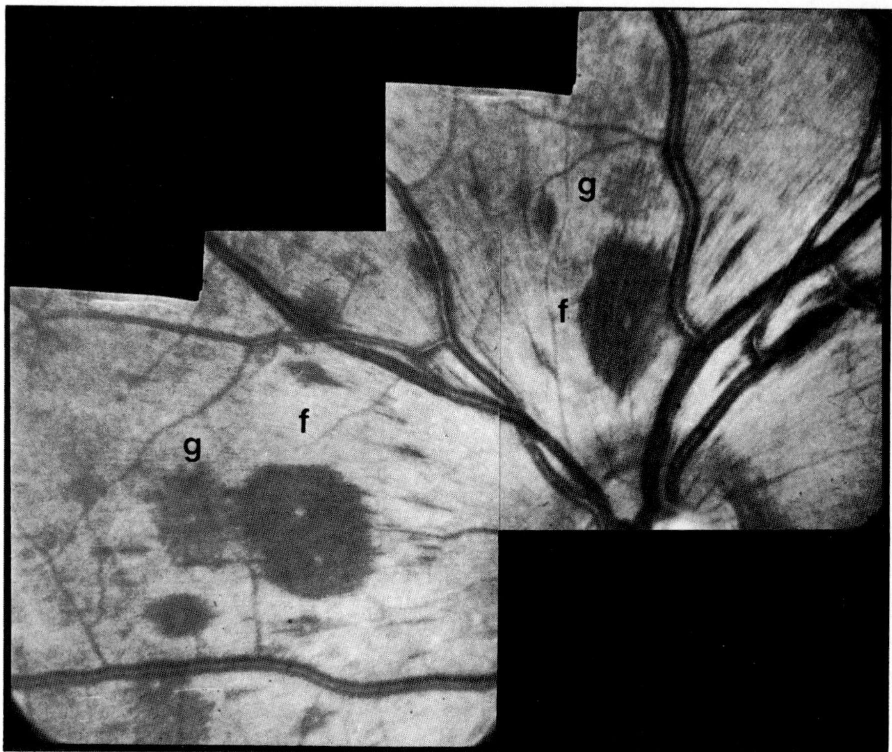

Fig. 1. Detail from Plate III. Typical configuration of flat intraretinal haemorrhages. *f*, flame-shaped haemorrhages of nerve fibre layer: linear and streak-like configurations, or patches with frayed borders, parallel to nerve fibre layer. *g*, granular haemorrhages of internal granular layer: nummular with dendritic borders and independent of nerve fibre layer

1. Haemorrhages with an outline shaped by the nerve fibre layer: They can be the smallest streaks, hardly visible by ophthalmoscopy; they can be spindle shaped, both ends always pointing along the direction of the nerve fibre layer; or they can form fringed patches, the fringes again oriented according to the nerve fibre layer. A common name is "flame-shaped", which well describes these haemorrhages confined to the fibrous layer.

2. Haemorrhages with an outline shaped by the inner granular layer: These round patches have dendritic or granular margins. Their density is lower than that of the flame-shaped haemorrhages, but more uniform.

Figure 2 illustrates the same two types of haemorrhages and beyond that a third element: round, deep red extravasations forming a hemispheric protuberance, with a brilliant light reflex on their summit. The outline is sharp if they are situated on unaffected retina, or less clearly marked if they are superimposed on a haemorrhage of the fibrous layer. This third group of hemispheric submembranacious haemorrhages — an extension of nerve fibre layer bleedings — will be discussed in Chap. III, Sect. A.3).

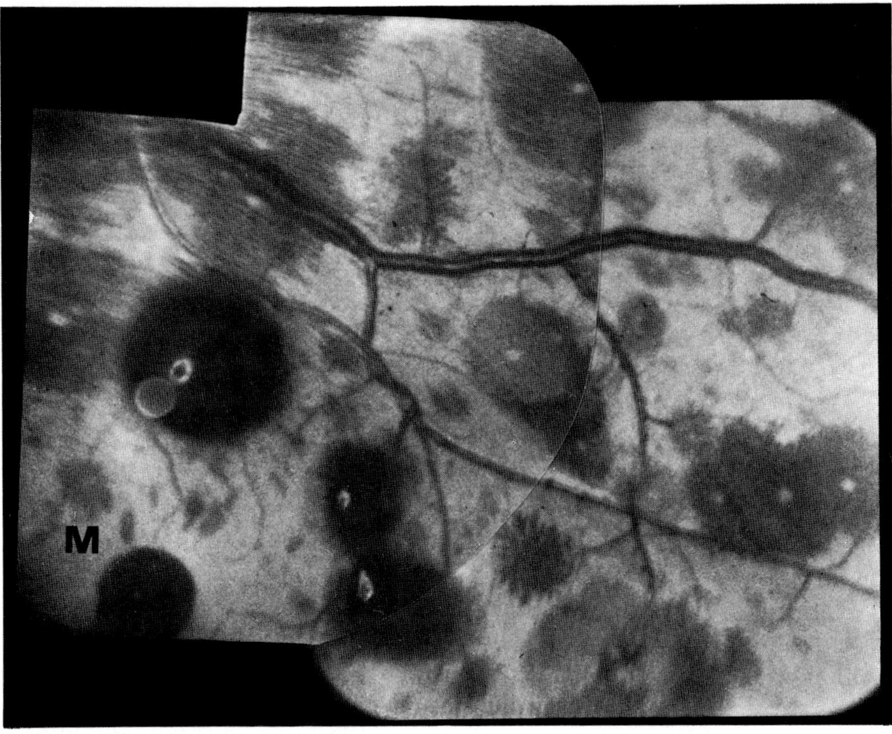

Fig. 2. Detail from Plate VII. Both types of flat haemorrhages again visible and, in addition, four dark red hemispheric submembranacious haemorrhages, with brillant white reflex on their summits. One of these (*M*) directly occupies fovea

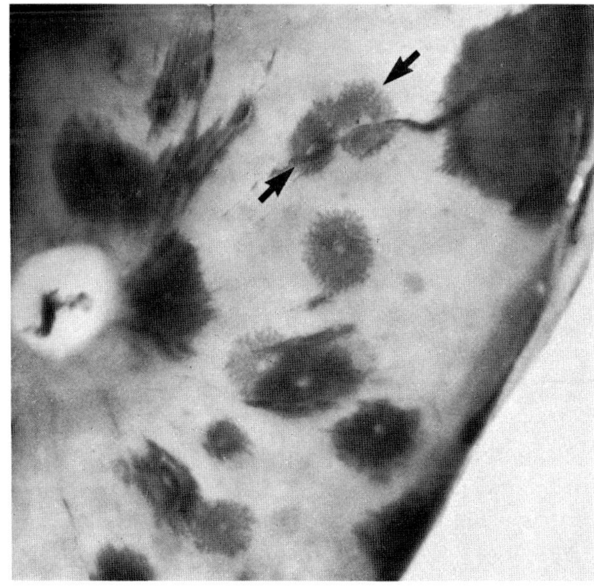

Fig. 3. Detail from Plate X. Flat haemorrhages in retina of a child having lived a few hours only. The appearance of these haemorrhages entirely corresponds to the in vivo observations. The two different types of haemorrhages indicated between *arrows* can be seen in the histologic section in Fig. 4

In order to correlate the two types of flat extravasations with the retinal layers, let us compare the in vivo retina to a post mortem specimen (Fig. 3). In this retina of a child that died a few hours after birth, the two types of intraretinal haemorrhages demonstrate essentially the same features as seen before. A section through adjacent extravasations of the two types demonstrates that they are strictly bound to two different retinal layers (Fig. 4). The haemorrhage in the nerve fibre layer is the one with the streaky or fringed outline, the other one in the internal granular layer has the dendritic or granular outline.

For further details, the five different haemorrhages indicated in Fig. 5 will be examined in particular. In anticipation of histologic documentation, it should be stated that the pale centre of the patchy haemorrhages consists of a thrombus of fibrin, occluding the vessel rupture.

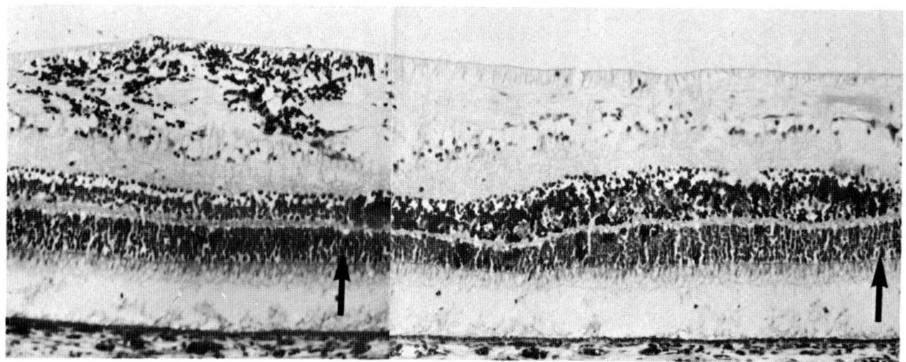

Fig. 4. Section through the two haemorrhages indicated in Fig. 3. The more centrally located haemorrhage of nerve fibre layer extends into layer of ganglion cells. The peripheral haemorrhage, of granular structure and dendritic outline, belongs to the internal granular layer, as marked between *arrows*. A few blood cells have also penetrated to the external granular layer. Paraffin, Goldner, x 200

1. Flame-Shaped Haemorrhages of the Nerve Fibre Layer

a) Histology

The ophthalmoscopic appearance demonstrating the relationsip of these haemorrhages to the nerve fibre layer has been illustrated before. The range of extent and localization will now be examined with the help of sections of the individual haemorrhages illustrated in Fig. 5.

The finest splinter- or streak-shaped haemorrhage (*a*) close to the disc consists of a few hundred red blood cells in a superficial stratum of the nerve fibre layer (Fig. 6). The cause of this bleeding, a capillary rupture, is not demonstrable in a paraffin section.

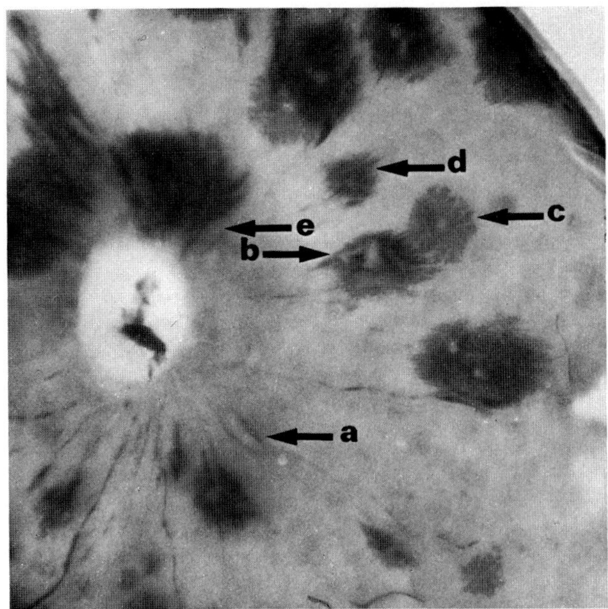

Fig. 5. Another detail from Plate X. The letters *a–e* correspond to the individual haemorrhages that will be analyzed in the following figures and in Figs. 31 and 32. Direction of *arrows* corresponds to direction of section

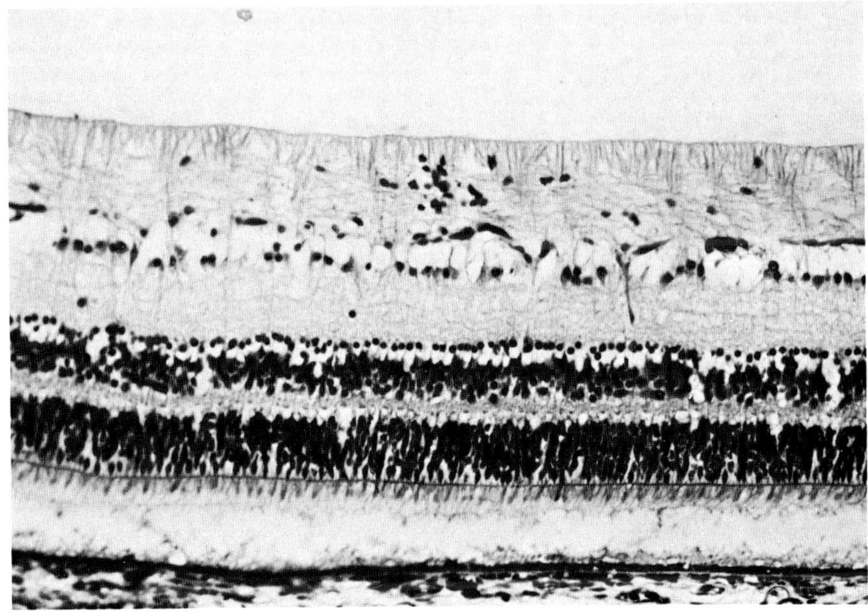

Fig. 6. Haemorrhage *a* from Fig. 5. This lightest degree of linear haemorrhage in the nerve fibre layer consists of a few red blood cells only. Paraffin, Goldner, x 230

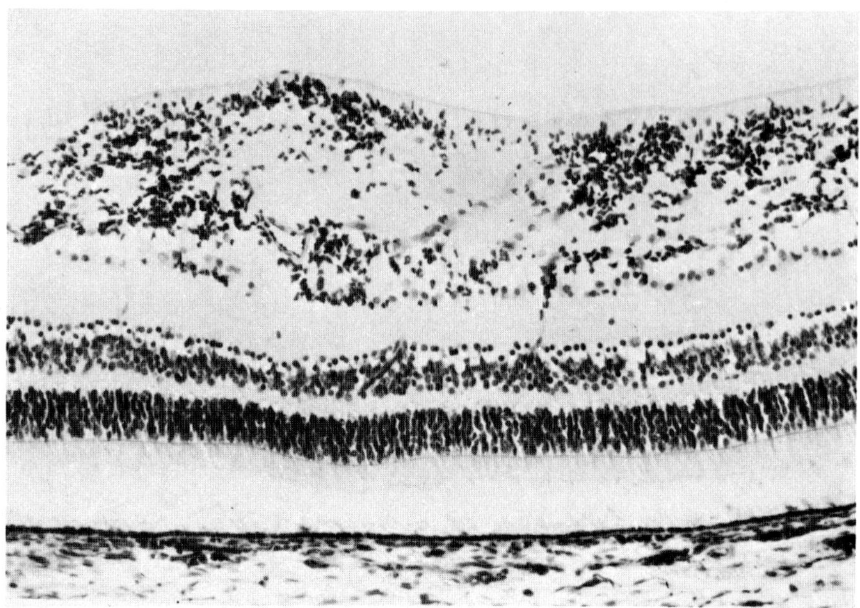

Fig. 7. Haemorrhage *b* from Fig. 5. This haemorrhage, shaped by the course of the nerve fibres, ranges from the internal limiting membrane to the internal plexiform layer, which is not penetrated. Close to disc, the high nerve fibre layer offers sufficient space for spread of hamorrhage. The light centre, also visible ophthalmoscicipally, corresponds to an area with few blood cells and a web-like deposit of fibrin. Paraffin, Goldner, x 200

The more extensive flame-shaped haemorrhage of the nerve fibre layer (*b*) shows the invasion of red blood cells from the base of the ganglion cell layer through the entire nerve fibre layer up to the internal limiting membrane (Fig. 7). The lighter centre of the haemorrhagic patch is caused by a loose packing of the blood cells surrounding the vessel rupture and by the occluding thrombus of fibrin. The rupture of the venule is situated within the nerve fibre layer itself. Haemorrhage *c* is situated in the ganglion cell layer and sections are demonstrated in Figs. 31 and 32 (p. 29).

The next haemorrhage (*d*), with macroscopically visible localization in the nerve fibre layer and histologically visible localization in the layer of ganglion cells (Figs. 8 and 9), was caused by a vessel rupture in this layer (Fig. 10). A dense clot of fibrin surrounded by finer web-like strands is in turn surrounded by less densely packed blood cells. Thus, looking onto the retina, a pale centre was visible here too.

Fig. 11 demonstrates a section through the superficial haemorrhage (*e*), passing over the margin of the disc. The continuity of the nerve fibres makes it easy to see how such haemorrhages can reach the centre of the disc without difficulty. This continuous overlapping is also illustrated by fundus photographs (Figs. 12 and 13). In addition these illustrations demonstrate how a greater number of extravasations may cover the posterior pole with confluent patches of blood in the superficial retina. Only the white fibrin thrombi indicate how many major vessel ruptures from the nerve fibre or ganglion cell layer are present.

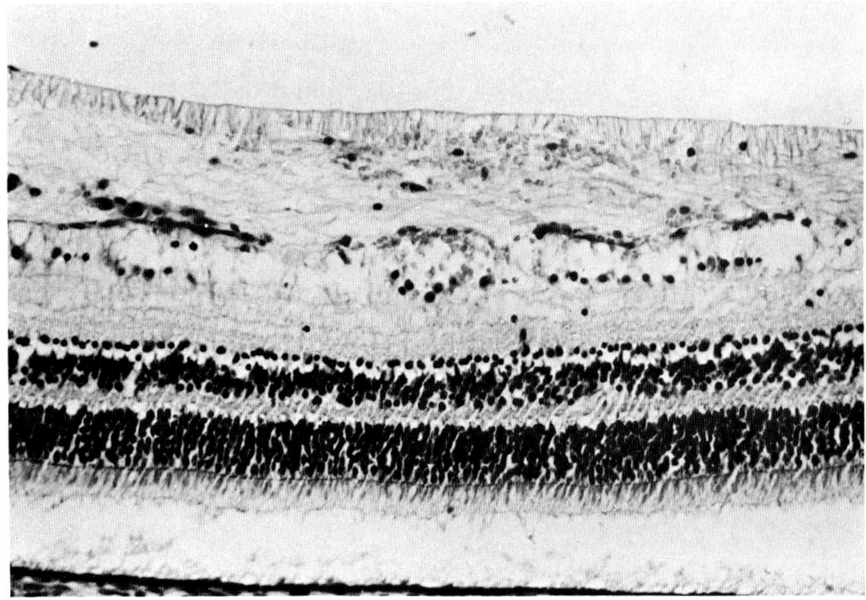

Fig. 8. Haemorrhage *d* from Fig. 5. Paraffin, haematoxilin-eosin, x 230

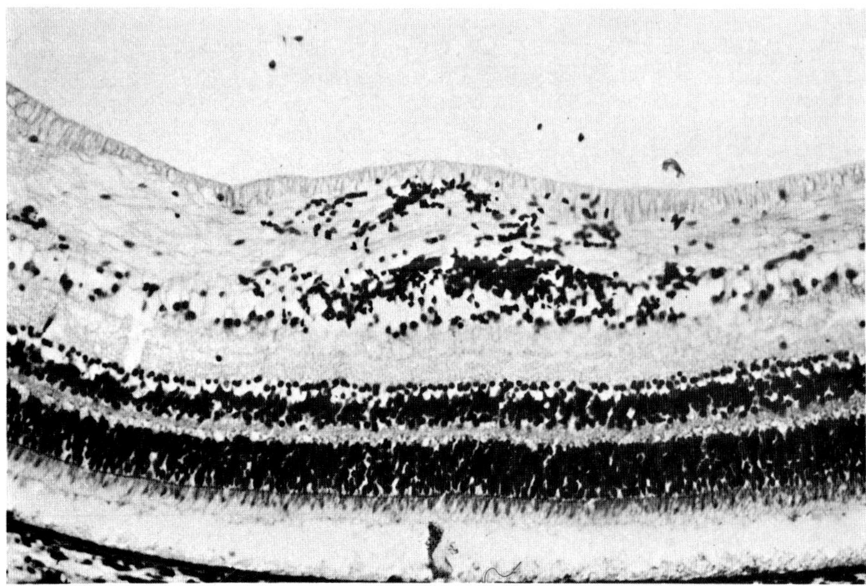

Fig. 9. Section through the same haemorrhage, *d*. This haemorrhage, outlined by the nerve fibre, originates from the layer of the ganglion cells. The relation of the normal cell population to the invading blood cells is best studied with different staining techniques. Paraffin, Goldner, x 180

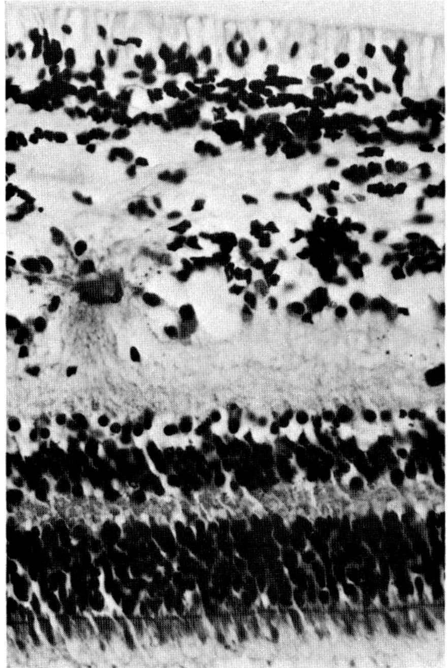

Fig. 10. Centre of haemorrhage *d* in another section. The source of bleeding is apparent through a clot of fibrin with finer strands in the ganglion cell layer. Paraffin, Goldner, x 500

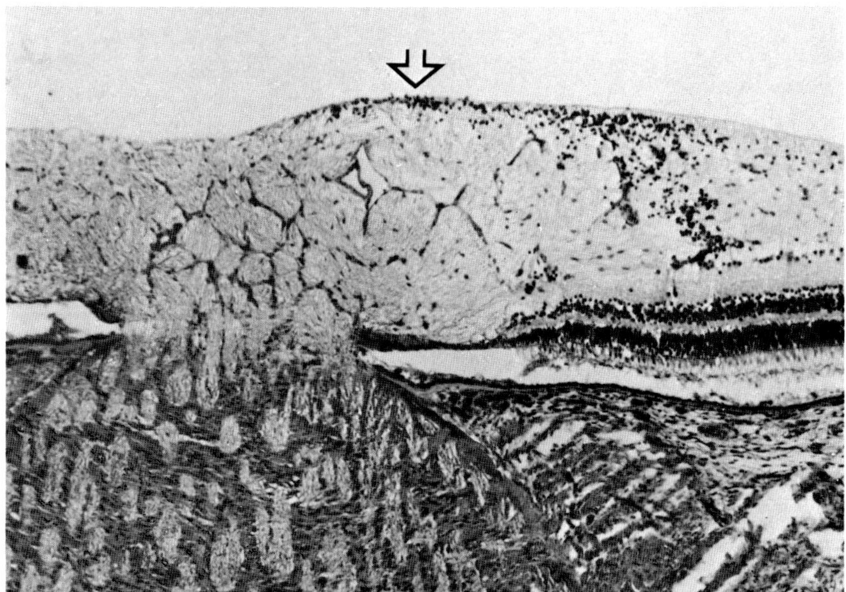

Fig. 11. Haemorrhage *e* from Fig. 5. Haemorrhage of nerve fibre layer close to border of disc. Blood cells spread from layer of ganglion cells to internal limiting membrane (*arrow*). Nerve fibres passing border of disc allow easy invasion in this direction. Paraffin, Goldner, x 140

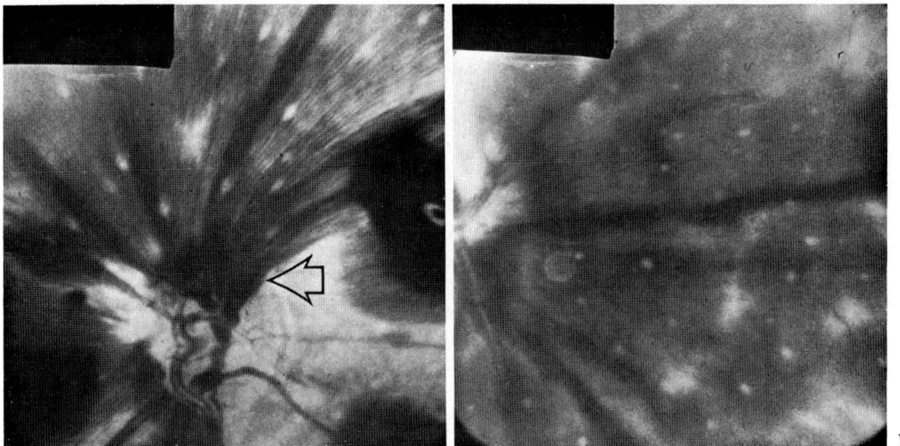

Figs. 12 and 13. Details from Plates VII and VIII. Confluent haemorrhages of nerve fibre layer close to disc, passing continuously over disc border (*arrow*)

b) Spread of Haemorrhages

Within the nerve fibre layer, there are two structures shaping and guiding the invasion of blood cells by providing virtual spaces: (1) the bundles of channels provided by the Müller cells for the nerve fibres and (2) perivascular spaces.

These types of spreading are demonstrated in Fig. 14 in a slightly immature retina. A venule is accompanied by superficial haemorrhages widening into a patch of bundles within the retina or along the vessel wall. Flat sections (Figs. 15 and 16) in the environment of this venule clearly show blood cells in their columnar orientation along the fascicular walls formed by Müller cells (cf. Fig. 35, p.31). This definite structure makes it easy to understand how smaller haemorrhages obtain the shape of a little streak or splinter whereas more extensive ones, covering many nerve fibre bundles, result in a patch with parallel fringes. Rupture of larger vessels will cause haemorrhages extending to the base of the ganglion cell layer but, according to our observations, not penetrating the very dense internal plexiform layer. Close to the macula and in the periphery, where the nerve fibre layer is rather flat, larger effusions create the hemispheric submembranacious haemorrhages discussed later.

The presence of real perivascular spaces is doubtful, according to electron-microscopic investigations (Hogan and Feeney, 1963). The vessels are surrounded by a collagenous network which can be extended by pathologic processes. This happens in the model of perinatal haemorrhages. The venule demonstrated in Figs. 3 and 4 is shown in two other sections in Figs. 17 and 18. In Fig. 17 the venule is cut traversing the granular haemorrhage illustrated in Fig. 4. The vessel walls are accompanied by an empty space, which must be regarded as an artefact. A parallel section (Fig. 18) demonstrates this same vessel closer to the very massive haemorrhage of the nerve fibre layer seen in the right upper corner of Fig. 4. Here, the blood cells have occupied this virtual space to the point that even the lumen of the venule is compressed. The vessel rupture creating this massive haemorrhage had occurred in a different smaller venule. Only the

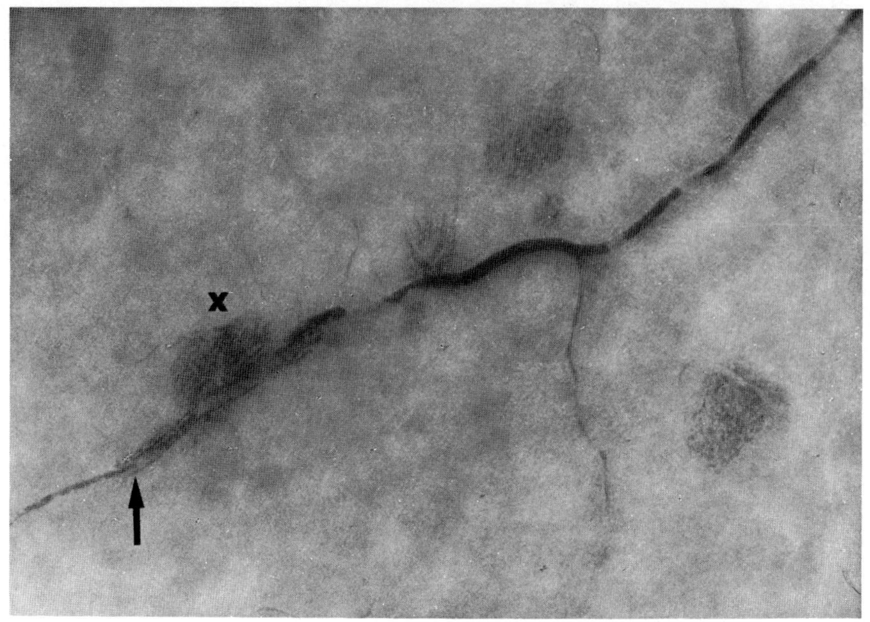

Fig. 14. Retina of immature infant, partly fixed with glutaraldehyde. Vein imcompletely filled with blood. Its walls partly delineated by blood cells invading virtual perivascular spaces (*arrow*). The flat haemorrhage (*x*) with parallel rows of blood cells is analyzed in flat sections in Figs. 15 and 16

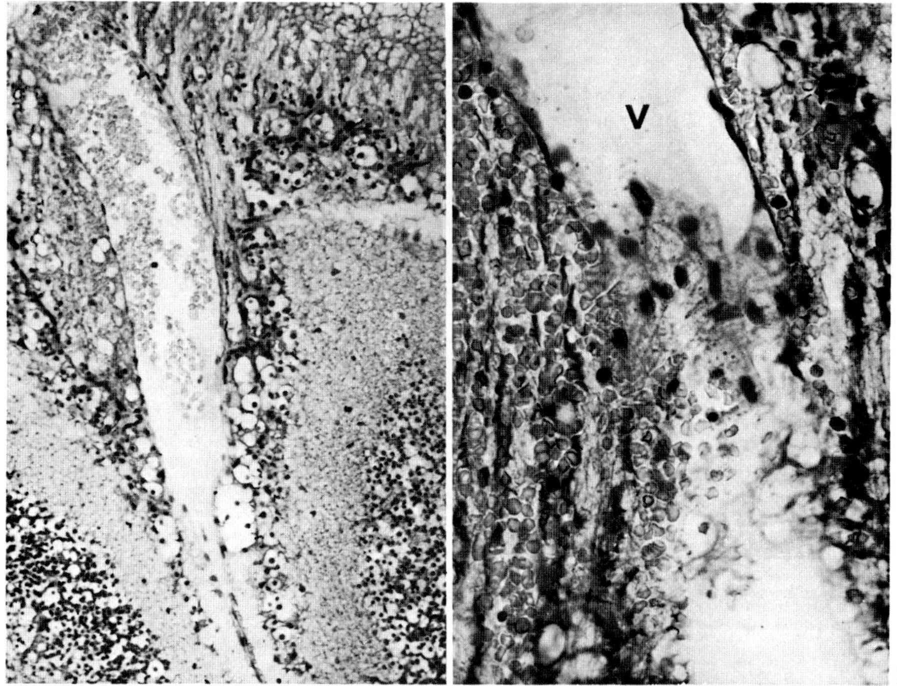

Figs. 15 and 16. Glutaraldehyde-fixed flat sections, paraffin, haematoxilin-eossin. Fig. 15. Nerve fibres passing in direction oblique to vein. *Right upper corner:* Honeycomb-like processes of Müller cells close to internal limiting membrane. *Lower corners:* Flat sections through internal granular layer. x 200
Fig. 16. Blood cells follow course of venous wall and strands of nerve fibres (*V*, venous lumen). x 500

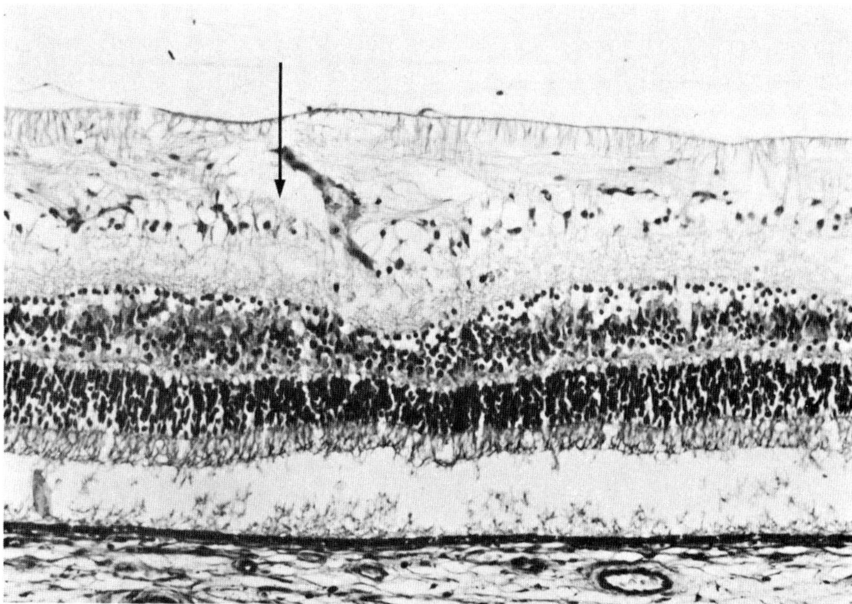

Fig. 17. Section parallel to Fig. 4, demonstrating venule passing over a haemorrhage of internal granular layer. Venule is surrounded by a loose cleavage space (*arrow*). Paraffin, haematoxilin-eosin, x 200

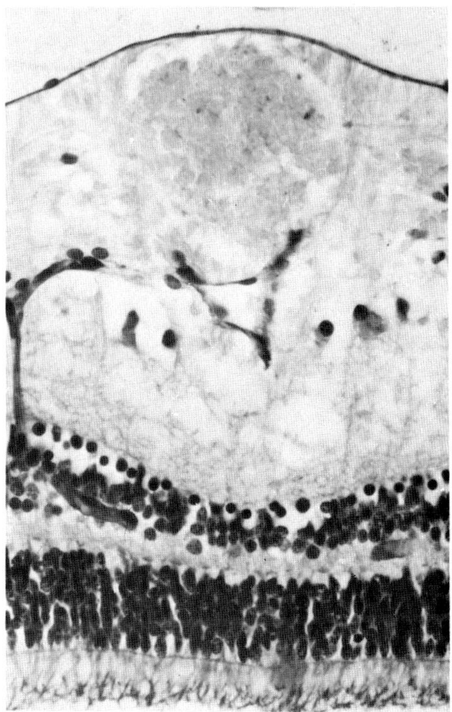

Fig. 18. More peripheral section through same venule. Blood cells from a huge confluent haemorrhage of nerve fibre layer have invaded virtual perivascular space, compressing venular lumen. Ophthalmoscopically this would produce the image of a fusiform dilatation of the vessel itself. Paraffin, PAS, x 500

easy accessibility of the virtual perivascular space caused its massive invasion. Within the fixed retina, too, this perivascular extension can be easily demonstrated (Fig. 19). Now the red blood cells appear light on a darker background. They accompany the vein far beyond the main haemorrhagic patch in the nerve fibre layer. In the original descriptions this feature was regarded as being a fusiform dilatation of the vein itself (Schleich, 1884; von Sicherer, 1907). This simulated fusiform vessel dilatation can be seen in Fig. 1 (the superior temporal artery) and Plates I, III and VII.

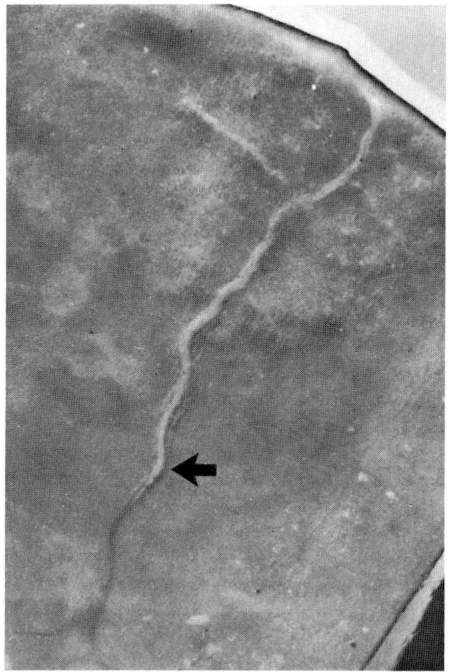

Fig. 19. Peripheral retina after fixation in formaldehyde. Blood cells brownish-white, moving along the nerve fibre bundles. Progression far outside original haemorrhagic area along vessel sheaths (*arrow*)

c) Source of Haemorrhages

As mentioned before, a white spot marks the centre of most of the haemorrhages of the nerve fibre layer and of the granular layer. This very characteristic white spot, not to be confused with the brillant light reflex on the top of the hemispheric submembramacious haemorrhages, is most precisely seen on fundus photographs. It is also clearly visible with a funduscope, though there is hardly ever a good description in the literature, and never a valuable interpretation. Meticulous serial sections prove that the white spot simply consists of a thrombus of fibrin, occluding the vessel rupture in single patches or the different sources of bleeding in confluent haemorrhages.

Figure 20 demonstrates this coagulum in the characteristic shape of an hour-glass. An intravascular portion is linked to an extravascular one by an isthmus which provides the actual occlusion of the ruptured vessel wall. This typical configuration is also easily demonstrable with flat preparations (Figs. 21—23). Again we see an intra- and

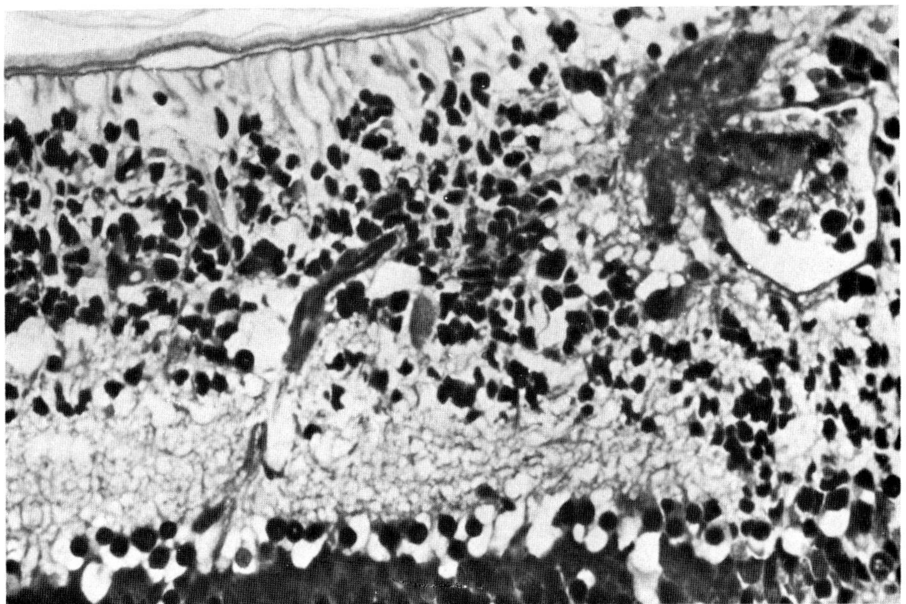

Fig. 20. Rupture of medium-sized venule. Defect of dilated vessel wall in *upper left quadrant.* Within lumen, mass of fibrin, with some enmeshed leucocytes. Outside vessel wall, rupture is surrounded by masses of densely packed fibrin. The two portions linked by an isthmus, which actually occludes vessel rupture. This is the centre of an extensive haemorrhage of the nerve fibre layer, the white fibrinous thrombus of which was easily visible macroscopically. Formalin-fixed and primarily paraffin-embedded section, reembedded in epon after postfixation with osmium tetroxide. Section 1.5 μm. Toluidine blue, x 930

an extra-vascular portion, connected by a constricted stem within the rupture site of the dilated venular wall. Venular dilatation is frequently visible, histologically and clinically.

While large fibrin thrombi of larger venules are easily demonstrable even in paraffin sections, the tracing of a fibrin becomes more and more difficult with decreasing vessel diameter. For example, the source of the haemorrhage of the inner granular layer demonstrated in Figs. 24 and 25 was a small venule. Its rupture was situated immediately at the junction of a capillary rising from the inner granular layer. Location of ruptures close to capillary anastomoses seems to be frequent. Paraffin sections are unable to disclose the ruptured vessel wall itself. For this purpose 1-μm sections of epon-embedded specimens have to be examined.

A characteristic example is presented in Figs. 26—28. In the neighbourhood of a fibrin clot the disruption of the dilated capillary can be detected. A similar capillary rupture was the source of the fibrin clot in Fig. 29, as in all other epon sections. This indicates that all haemorrhages are caused by rhexis and that no connection to diapedesis can be found (as had been discussed in the literature).

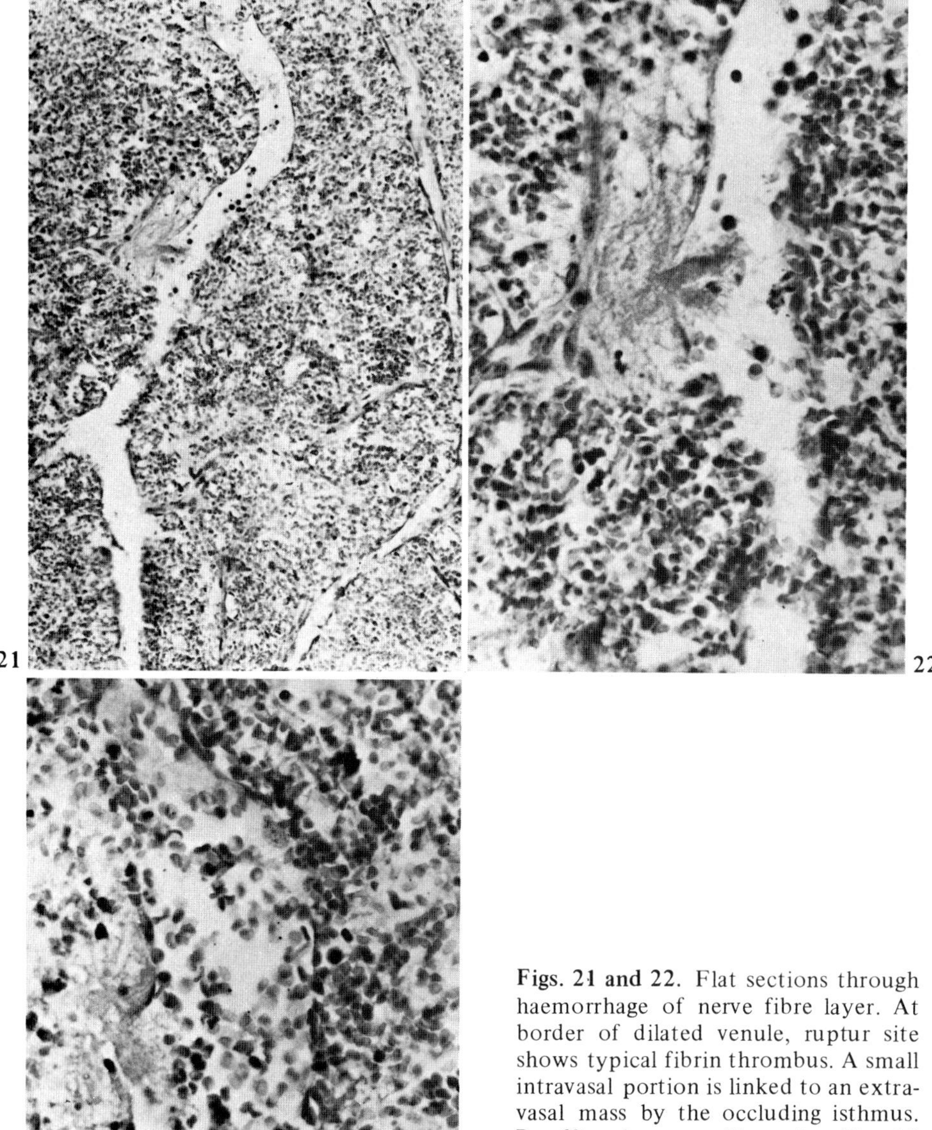

Figs. 21 and 22. Flat sections through haemorrhage of nerve fibre layer. At border of dilated venule, ruptur site shows typical fibrin thrombus. A small intravasal portion is linked to an extravasal mass by the occluding isthmus. Paraffin, haematoxilin-eosin. Fig 21 x 200, Fig. 22 x 500

Fig.. 23. Another flat section of the peripheral retina, with a typical fibrin thrombus: An intra- and extravasal portion, occluding the rupture of the dilated venule. Paraffin, haematoxilin-eosin, x 500

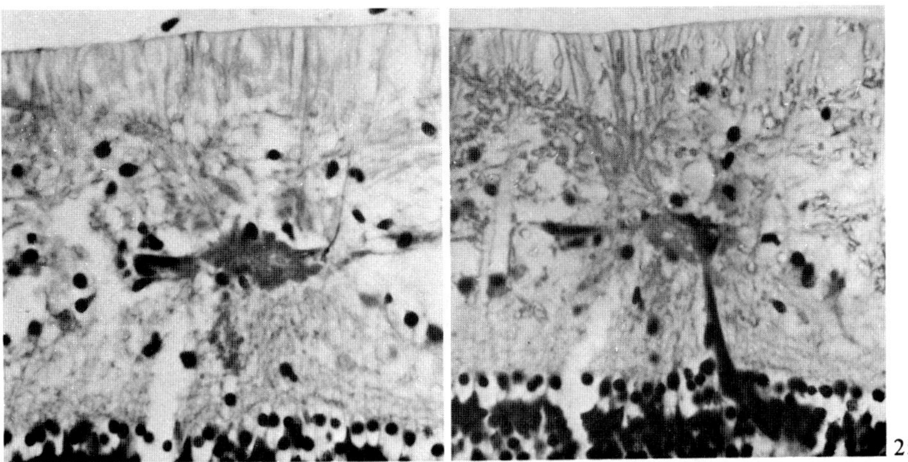

Figs. 24 and 25. Fibrin clot at the rupture site of small venule; adjacent sections of 10 μm. At a capillary junction emanating from the internal granular layer, a rupture has occurred, of which the fibrin thrombus is visible. Erythrocytes spread into the layer of ganglion cells and nerve fibres.

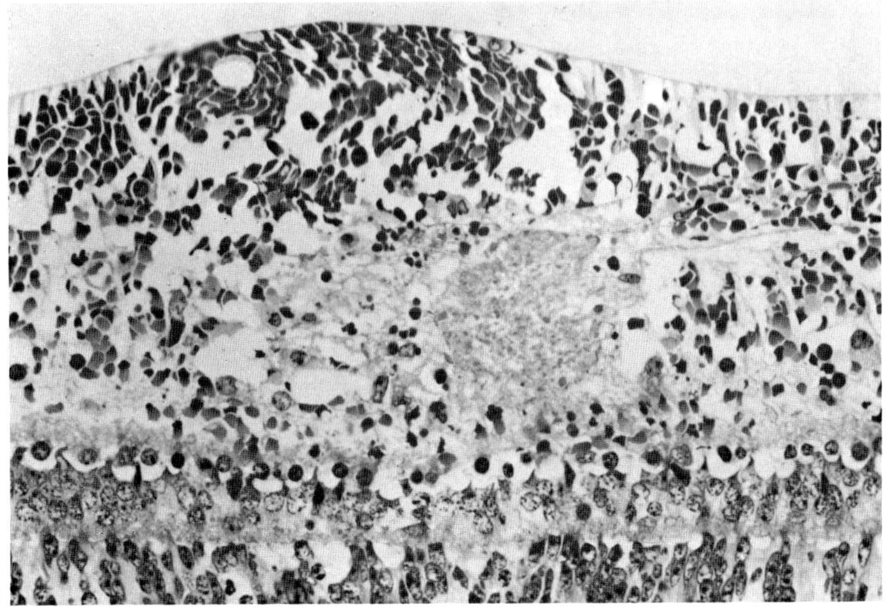

Figs. 26, 27 and 28. Adjacent sections from capillary rupture of equatorial retina. Blood cells have collected between nerve fibres and extended Müller cell processes. Close to vessel, mass of fibrin (Fig. 26) behind which rupture itself is seen (Fig. 27, c.f. p. 26). In Fig. 28, *arrow* indicates very delicate outline of vessel, which is interrupted from 7 to 9 o'clock. Epon, toluidine blue; Figs. 26 and 27, x 500; Fig. 28, x 1040

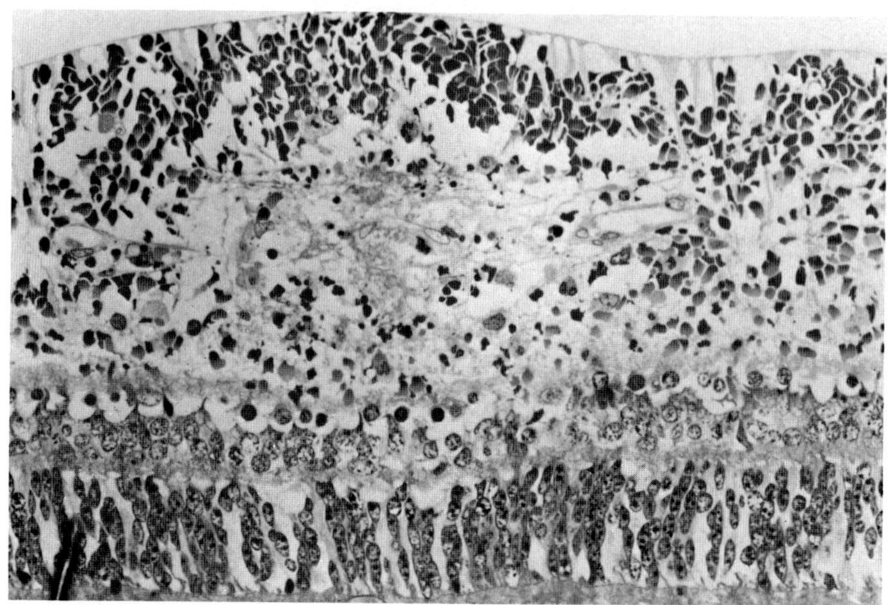

Fig. 27

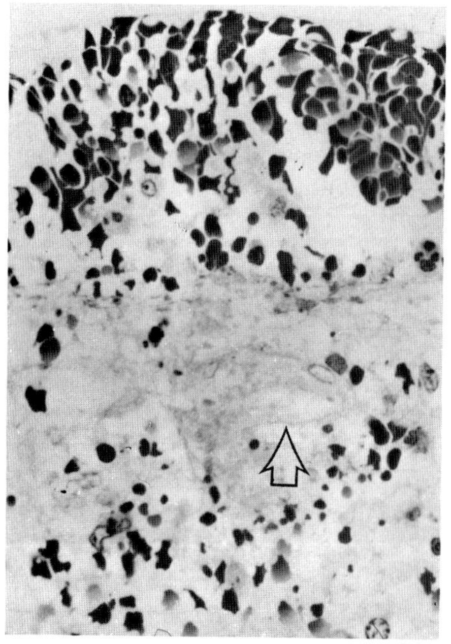

Fig. 28

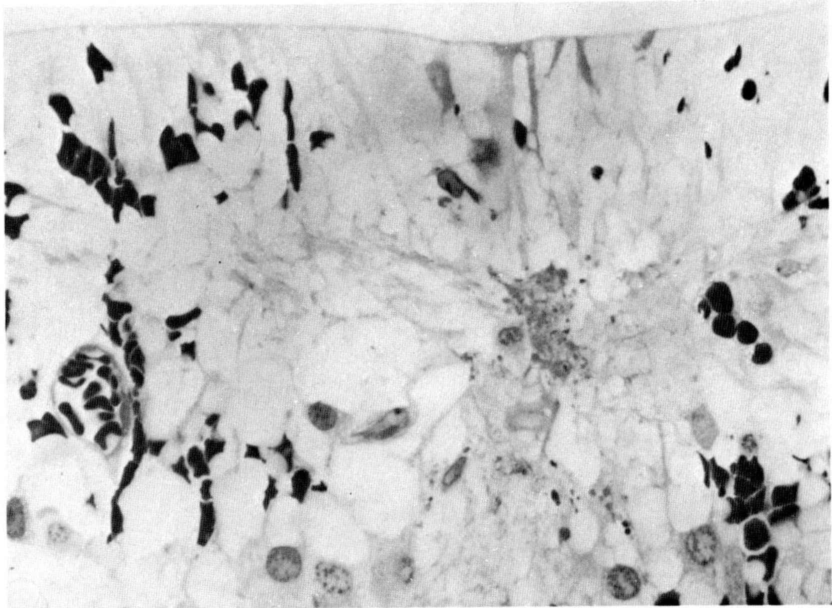

Fig. 29. Very small collection of fibrin at site of capillary rupture, surrounded by area with very few blood cells. Epon, toluidine blue, x 800

2. Granular Haemorrhages of the Internal Granular Layer

a) Histology

Figure 4 demonstrates that a second type of flat haemorrhage occurs in the internal granular layer. This localization causes the different appearance of these haemorrhages. With different staining methods the arrangement of red blood cells in their relation to the nuclei of this layer is very well visible, much more so than in black and white photographs. Figure 30 tries to demonstrate the result of Goldner staining of a section with two layers of haemorrhages: A haemorrhage of the nerve fibre layer extends from the ganglion cells to the internal limiting membrane and has no connection with the haemorrhage of the internal granular layer. Both haemorrhages are caused by vessel ruptures in their own stratum.

Two other examples are demonstrated in Fig. 31 by haematoxylin-eosin staining and in Fig. 32 by PAS staining. The orientation of blood cells in small vertical columns is visible (cf. Fig. 30). This columnar arrangement is even better visible in Fig. 33, an epon-embedded specimen of the retina of an immature infant. A flat section (Fig. 34) also shows how the red blood cells appear in clusters interspersed between the cellular elements of the internal granular layer.

A schematic drawing from Hogan et al. (1971) shows how the blood cells can fill in virtual spaces in the internal nuclear layer (Fig. 35). The typical arrangement of red blood cells in this layer in vertical columns or, in the flat section, in small clusters, easily explains the dendritic outline and the rather uniform density of these haemorrhages.

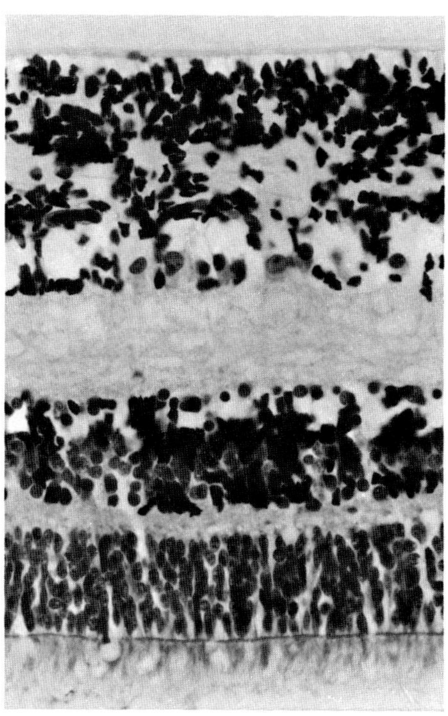

Fig. 30. Overlapping flat haemorrhages from different sources of bleeding. Goldner staining with light staining of nuclei to demonstrate clusters of red blood cells in internal granular layer. Internal plexiform layer is free of blood cells. Haemorrhage of nerve fibre layer extends from ganglion cells to internal limiting membrane. Paraffin, Goldner, x 500

b) Spread of Haemorrhages

Unlike the case with the more superficial effusions, the space for further invasion remains restricted for granular haemorrhages. The dendritic plexus of the internal plexiform layer, with its large number of tight junctions (Dowling and Boycott, 1965), forms a dense barrier against the penetration of blood cells.

The external plexiform layer is not so densely structured and thus allows penetration into the external nuclear layer, as demonstrated in Figs. 31 and 32. Penetrations of the external limiting membrane were not observed in this series, but they have been described in the literature. But even the dense internal plexiform layer can be penetrated. Figure 36 shows a few red blood cells pressed into this layer above the centre of bleeding of the inner granular layer. A complete rupture of the internal plexiform layer is illustrated by Fig. 37 and Plate XII. Here the blood cells have invaded a limited area of the inner nuclear layer and then have burst into the superficial layers. With this explosive infiltration cellular elements from the inner nuclear layer have been transported up to the nerve fibre layer. The gross aspect of this unusual and destructive haemorrhage is seen in Fig. 3 (p. 13). In this case the superficial effusion within the nerve fibre layer hides the source of the bleeding. Ophthalmoscopically, this haemorrhage would have been suspected to have originated from the nerve fibre layer.

In general, though, haemorrhages from the internal granular layer tend to be more uniform and light red in colour because of their homogeneity. If they spread out into other layers, it will be mainly to the outer nuclear layer.

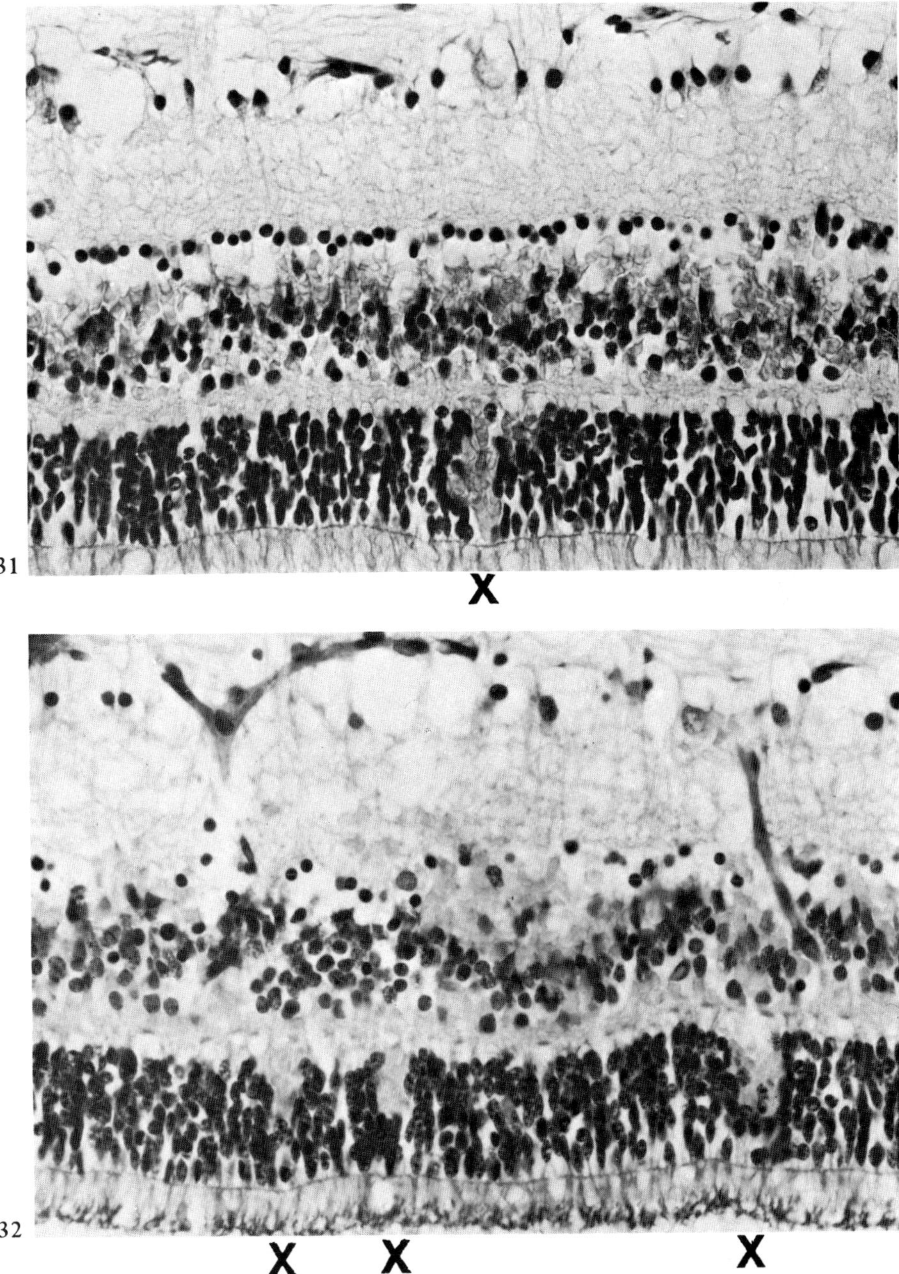

Figs. 31 and 32. Haemorrhages of internal granular layer (*c* from Fig. 5) demonstrated with different staining techniques. Here clusters of blood cells invade external graunlar layer and reach external limiting membrane (*x*). Haematoxilin-eosin, PAS, Fig. 31 x 450 and Fig. 32 x 500

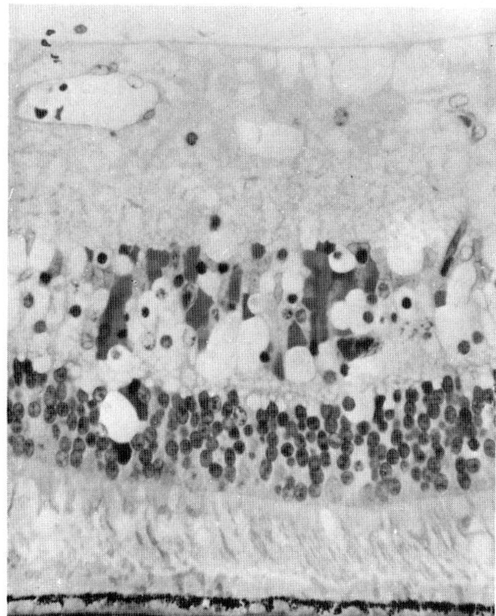

Fig. 33. Retina of immature infant. Haemorrhage of internal granular layer shows clusters of red blood cells pushing aside cells of this layer. Glutaraldehyde, epon, toluidine blue, x 400

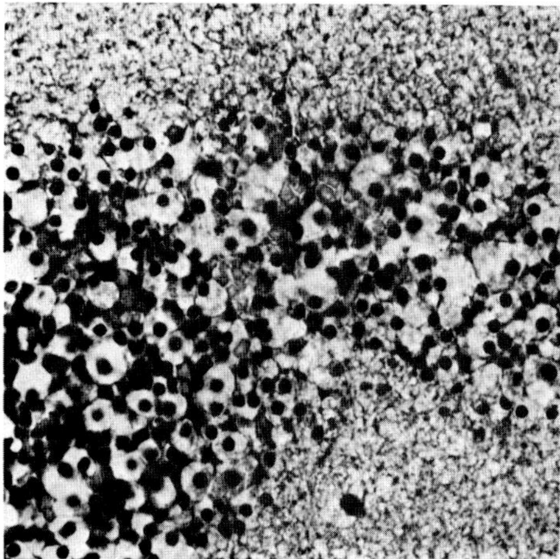

Fig. 34. Flat section through small haemorrhage of internal granular layer. Red blood cells arranged in clusters among cells of this layer. Glutaraldehyde, epon, toluidine blue, x 500

c) Source of Haemorrhages

The usually constant size of the haemorrhage from the internal granular layer is explained by the fairly uniform calibre of vessels that can cause this bleeding. The only vessels reaching this layer are capillaries, whereas in the nerve fibre layer extravasations can be caused by a wide range of vessels from capillaries to larger venules. Accordingly we can only expect capillary ruptures within the internal nuclear layer. Figure 38 shows a typical fibrin clot forming the white centre of such an extravasation. As in most of the haemorrhages of the nerve fibre layer the thrombus is surrounded by a seemingly empty zone with few blood cells. In some paraffin sections no clot of fibrin is visible, although it is present in epon-embedded material.

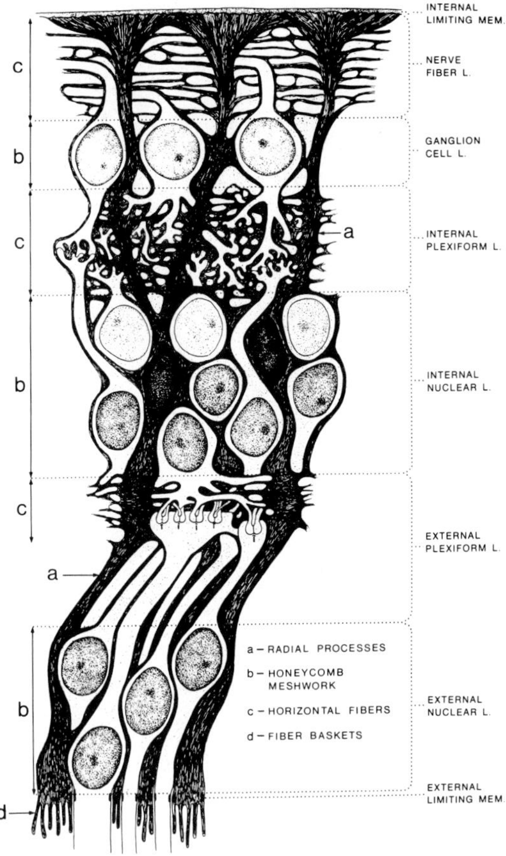

Fig. 35. Schematic drawing of Müller cells and retinal layers influenced by their structure (Hogan et al., 1977)

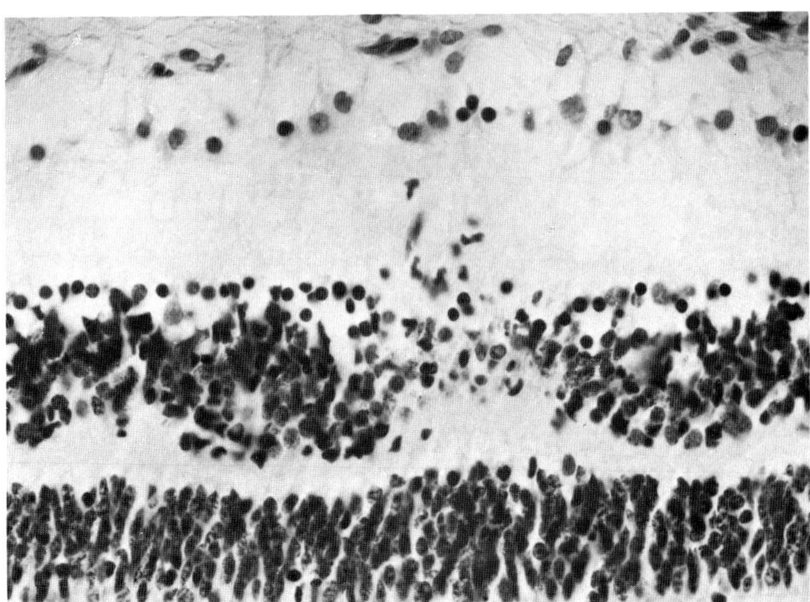

Fig. 36. Centre of another capillary rupture of internal granular layer with red blood cells penetrating to this layer. Fewer blood cells in the centre, but a few have even penetrated into the internal plexiform layer. Paraffin, Goldner, x 500

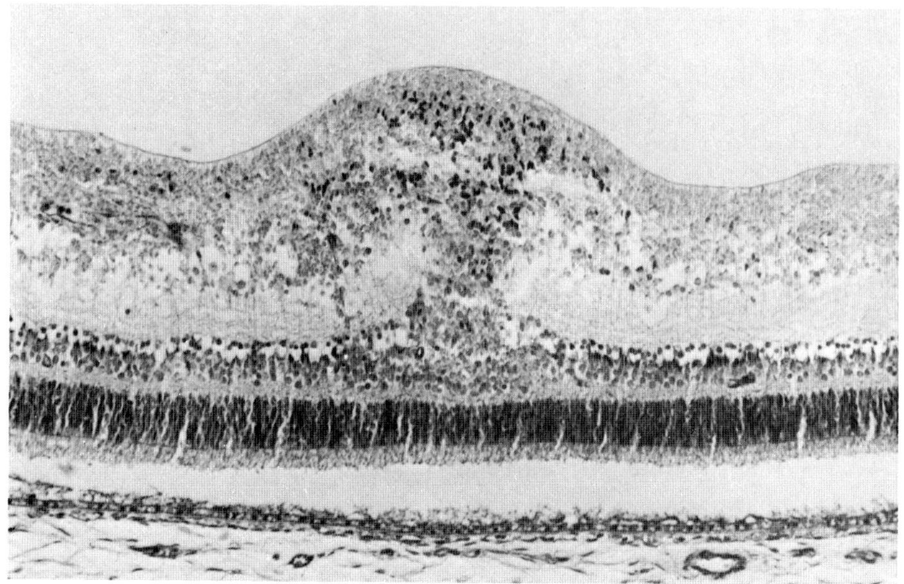

Fig. 37. Haemorrhage of internal nuclear layer penetrating into superficial layers. Vessel rupture not demonstrable in this PTAH staining. Blood cells have invaded only a limited area of internal nuclear layer and then have burst through internal plexiform layer, thus passing from ganglion cell layer to internal limiting membrane. With this definitely destructive eruption, nerve elements from the internal nuclear layer have been transported into the superficial layers (cf. Plate XII). Paraffin, PTAH, x 200

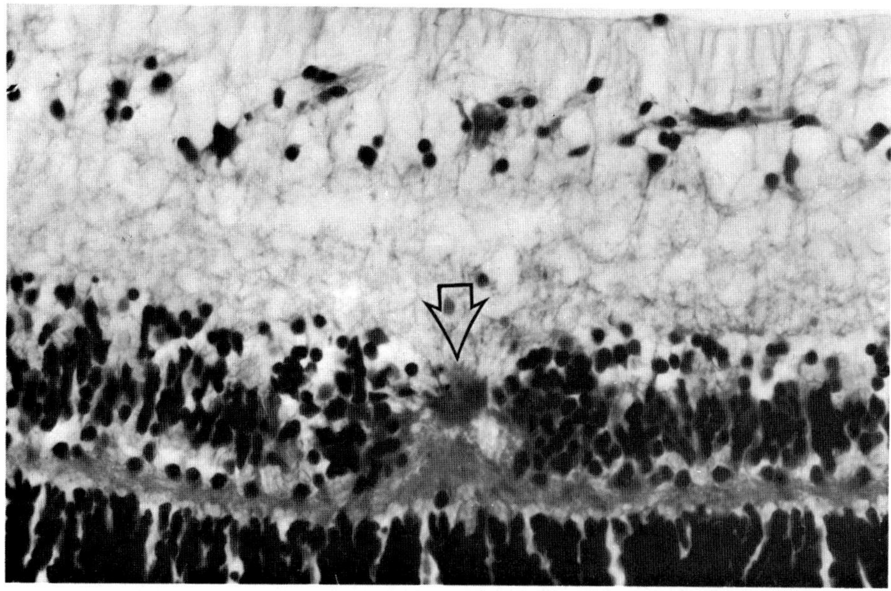

Fig. 38. Capillary rupture in centre of haemorrhage of internal granular layer. In paraffin section capillary itself not demonstrable, but clot of fibrin with surrounding halo of a few blood cells corresponds to white centre of such a haemorrhage (*arrow*). Goldner, x 500

3. Hemispheric Submembranacious Haemorrhages

a) Ophthalmoscopy

This third type is different from the two flat types of retinal effusions described and causes an elevation of the retinal surface. This suggested to some authors that they were subretinal; more frequently they are called preretinal. Actually they are still confined to the retina itself. What we see is a dark red elevation with a borderline which may be sharp, as in Fig. 39, or less distinct (Fig. 2) if a haemorrhage in the nerve fibre layer disguises this contour (Plates I, II, V, VI, VII, VIII and IX). The brillant light reflex on top of the elevation, wandering with the movement of the ophthalmoscope, is very typical. This must not be confused with the white fibrin thrombus visible in the flat haemorrhages. Sometimes a white clot can be seen at the border and represents the eccentric original source of bleeding (Fig. 40; Plates I, VII and IX). Normally this is hidden under the compact aggregation of blood cells.

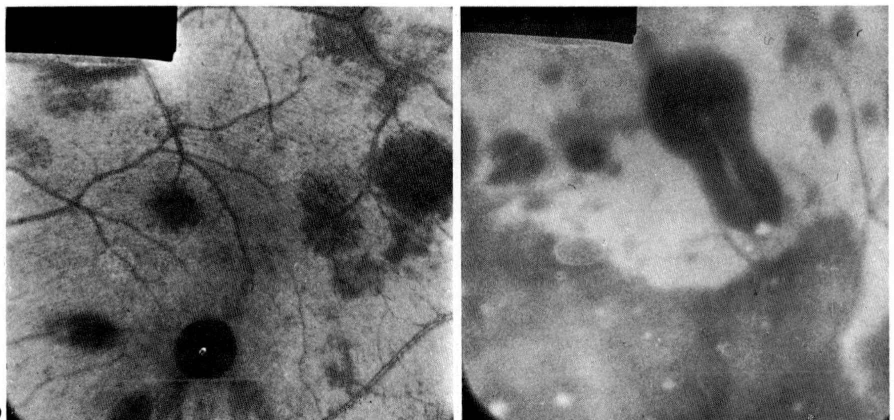

Fig. 39. Detail from Plate V. Macular haemorrhage with clearly outlined, hemispheric protuberance. Brillant light reflex of detached internal limiting membrane. Other granular and flame-shaped haemorrhages in vicinity. Small flame-shaped haemorrhage at 7 o'clock seems to contain vessel rupture, from which submembranacious haemorrhage originated. Follow-up cf. Fig. 63, p. 131

Fig. 40. Detail from Plate IX. Confluent superficial haemorraghes of nerve fibre layer with multiple fibrin thrombi. Fovea is covered by submembranacious haemorrhage in the shape of a calabash. White spot at inferior border occludes original vessel rupture from which detachment of internal limiting membrane reached macula (cf. Plate I with a very similar situation. Follow-up cf. Fig. 64, p. 132)

This type of haemorrhage tends to be concentrated around the macula and normally occurs with other severe extravasations. If the fovea is affected it is only with this type. At times a rather isolated submembranacious haemorrhage can occur in the mid-periphery as can be seen in Plate II. In the literature this localization is known practically only from post mortem specimens. Figure 41 shows such a shadow-casting

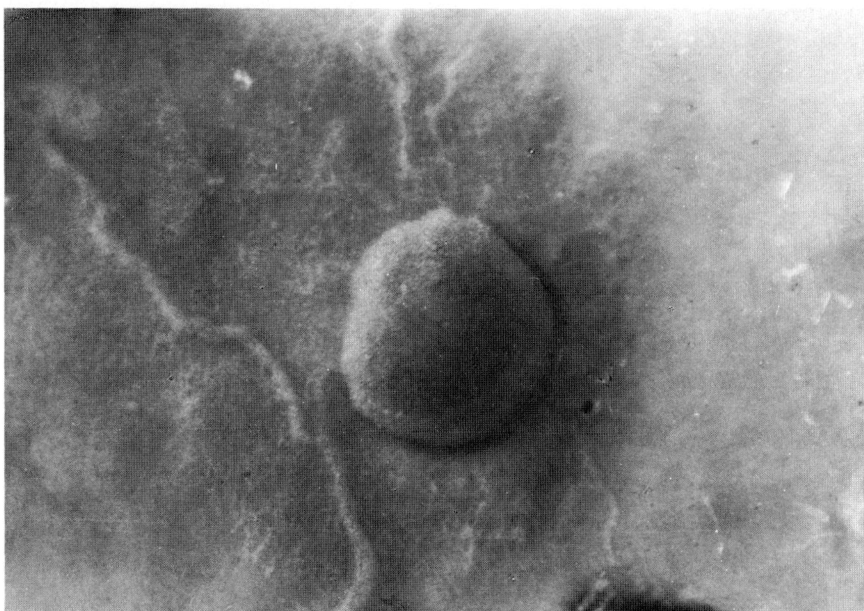

Fig. 41. Submembranacious haemorrhage of 1-mm diameter. Peripheral retina fixed in formaldehyde. Hemispheric submembranacious haemorrhage bulges over venule with limited extravasations into surroundings. Exaggerated steepness of margins is an artefact of fixation (loose packing of blood cells under detachment of internal limiting membrane)

elevation of the mid-periphery in the fixed retina. The superficial reflex seen in vivo is not present in the fixed state. The very steep elevation at the border is an artefact. This submembranacious haemorrhage is the continuation of the patchy haemorrhage of the superficial retinal layers, which also accompanies the veins, as demonstrated in Fig. 19 (p. 22).

b) Histology

Sections through the haemorrhage shown in Fig. 41 demonstrate very particular features (Fig. 42). Detached and highly elevated, the internal limiting membrane forms the borderline of this haemorrhage adjoining the vitreous body. The mass of red blood cells consists of two parts. The inferior lenticular part remains densely packed, even with fixation. The superior part, crescentic in the section, seems to be less densely packed, an artefact of the preparation. At a higher magnification (Figs. 43 and 44) we see that these masses of blood overlie an otherwise typical haemorrhage of the nerve fibre and ganglion layer. The great difference now is that definite tissue lesions have occurred. The flat haemorrhages described before had only invaded the easily accessible virtual spaces between the nerve fibres, or the ganglion cells, along the vessel sheaths, or between the cells of the inner nuclear layer. All these extravasations are not very destructive (the rupture through the inner plexiform layer was mentioned as a rare exception).

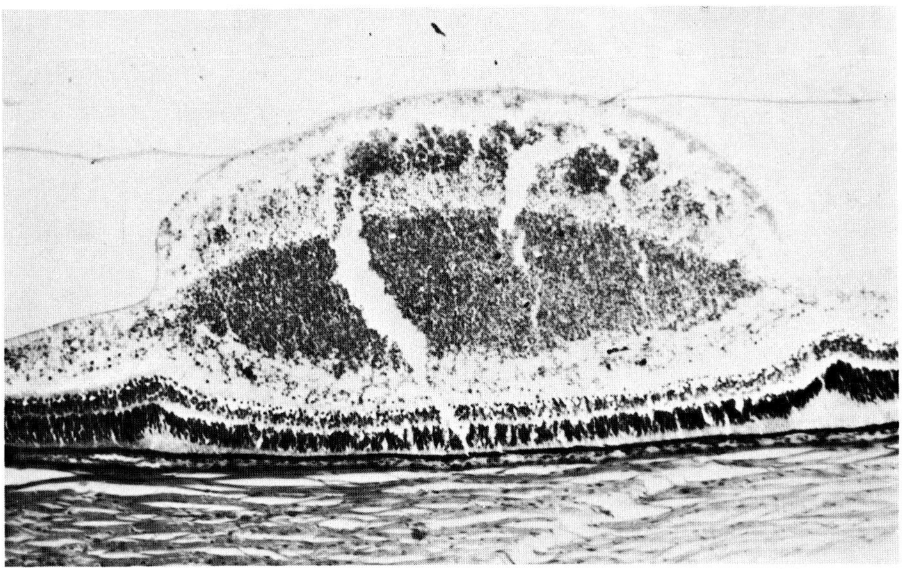

Fig. 42. Section of submembranacious haemorrhage from Fig. 41. Haemorrhage consists of two parts: A densely packed one within the upper part of the over-burdened nerve fibre layer and, superimposed, a loosely packed mass of blood cells, limited by the internal limiting membrane. Paraffin, haematoxilin-eosin, x 90

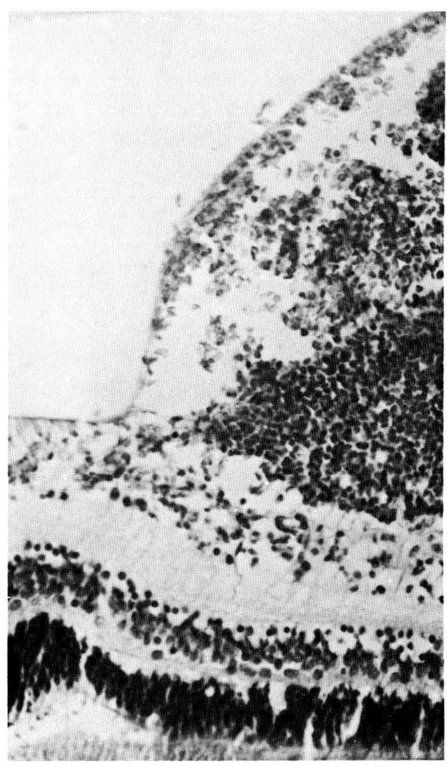

Figs. 43 and 44. Margins of submembranacious haemorrhage from Fig. 42. Sections demonstrate how internal limiting membrane is elevated and finally detached from connection to Müller cells. Two portions of haemorrhage clearly visible. Fig. 43, haematoxilin-eosin, x 200; Fig. 44, PAS, x 500

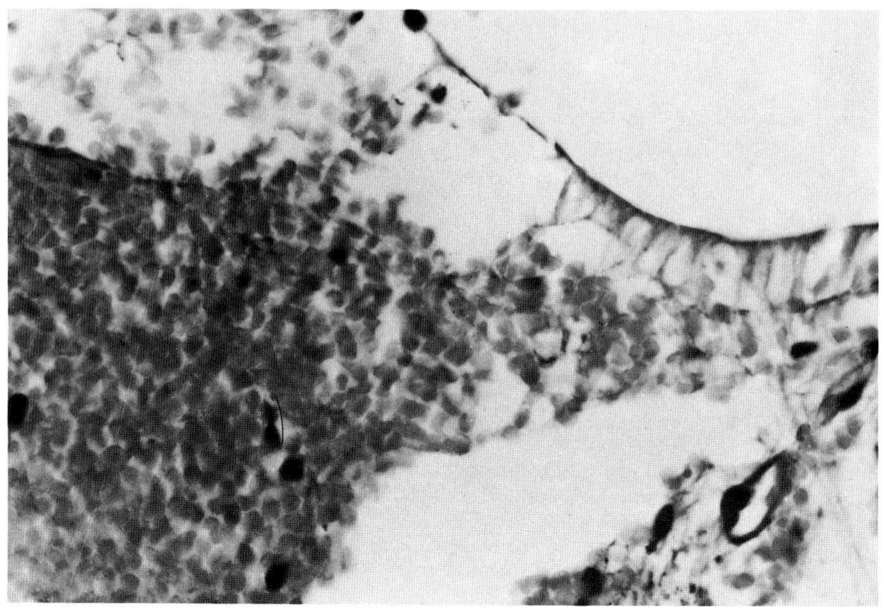

Fig. 44 (legend see p. 35)

These hemispheric haemorrhages have elevated the internal limiting membrane, by lifting it from its connection with the Müller cells (cf. Fig. 35, p. 31). The Müller cell processes obviously can stand a certain amount of stretching, as demonstrated in Figures 26,27 and 28. Figure 44 shows how they finally relinquish their palm-like connections (Rohen, 1969) with the internal limiting membrane. This membrane itself proves to be very resistent and normally will withstand further invasion. When no rupture of the internal limiting membrane occurs, the term "preretinal" haemorrhages is not correct; the haemorrhages are still confined to the retinal tissue.

The basic vessel rupture, with its fibrin thrombus directly on top of the inner plexiform layer, is demonstrated in Figures 45, 46 and 47. Also in this haemorrhage, the typical structure is visible with a densely packed lower mass of blood cells, and loosely packed upper mass of blood cells. The real difference between these two layers is hidden by the blood cells themselves in normal stainings. A selective staining of nuclei only (Fig. 48) proves that the inferior part consists of blood cells still remaining within a distorted retina. The superficial layer lies above all cellular elements of the retina but under the elevated internal limiting membrane.

The dynamic mechanism for this type of haemorrhage must be as follows: The amount of blood escaping from a larger venule exceeds the quantity which can invade the virtual spaces within the retina. This would occur in the areas with a thin nerve fibre layer, as in the macular area and in the periphery. Thus the connections of the Müller cells with the internal limiting membrane are stretched and finally torn, and, similar to a dissecting aneurysm, the haemorrhage will lift this membrane. The dense vascularization surrounding the macula provides many possible sources for bleeding,

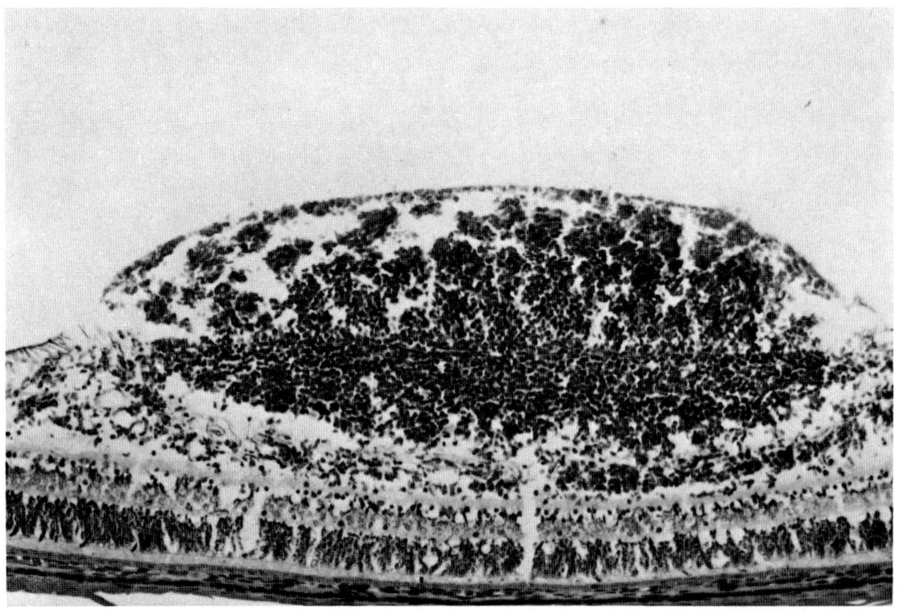

Figs. 45, 46 and 47. Submembranacious
haemorrhage of retinal periphery. Paraffin, haematoxilin-eosin.
Fig. 45. Typical composition of two
portions. x 200

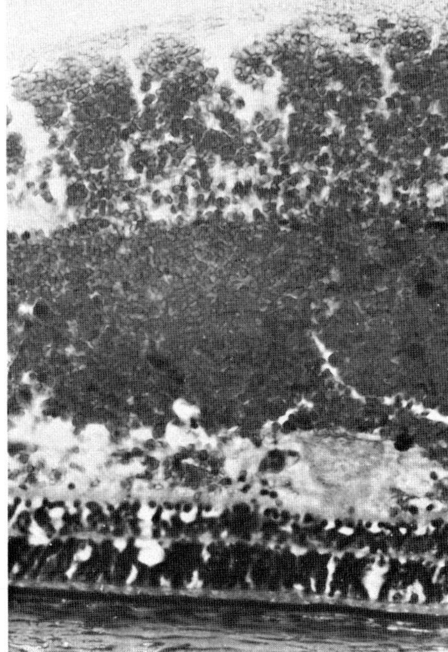

Fig. 46. Central part of haemorrhage
with fibrin thrombus at internal plexiform layer. x 400

but little space within the nerve fibre layer. This leads to the spread under the limiting
membrane, and sometimes right into the fovea. No foveal haemorrhage, of course, can
have its origin in this avascular area itself.

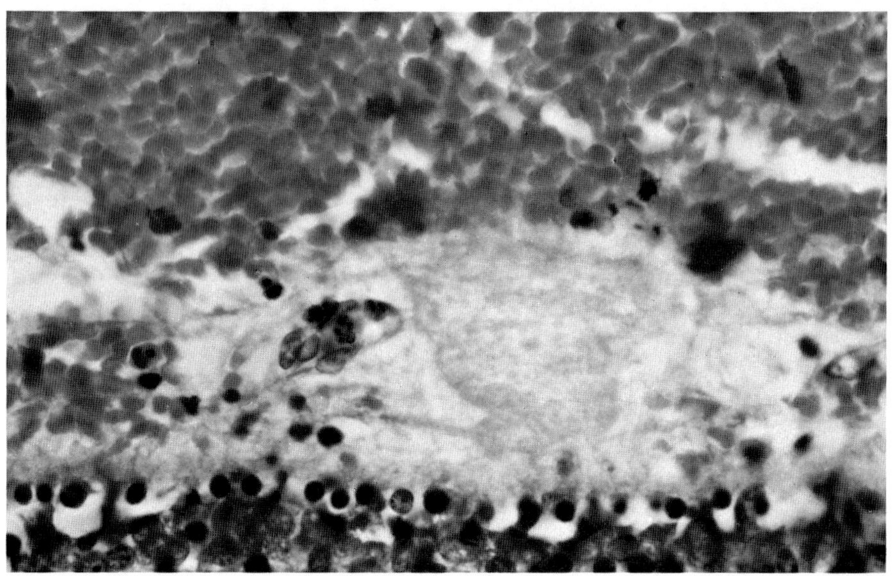

Fig. 47. Detail from Fig. 46. Fibrin thrombus at site of vessel rupture. x 1000

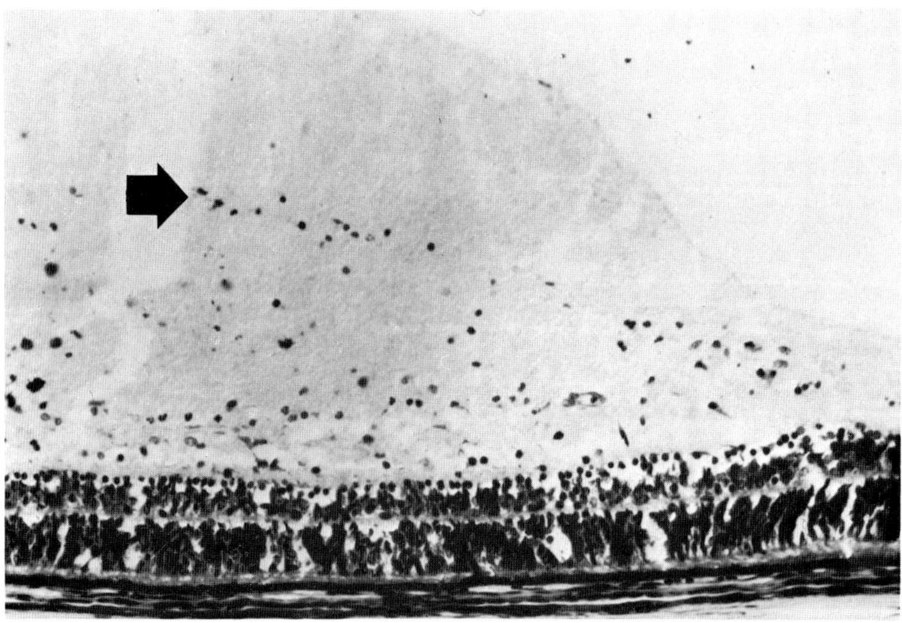

Fig. 48. Staining of nuclei with cresyl violet. Superficial layer under internal limiting membrane contains red blood cells only. Inferior portion contains blood cells expanding superficial retinal layers from ganglion cells to nerve fibres. *Arrow* indicates border of these portions. Paraffin, cresyl violet, x 260

4. Discussion

Three years after the first clinical description of perinatal retinal haemorrhages, Ulrich (1884) reported on the histologic aspect. He found haemorrhages most frequently in the nerve fibre layer, but also in the ganglion cell layer and the internal granular layer. The most thorough and detailed examination up to now is the excellent publication of Naumoff from St. Petersburg (1890). He reports on 47 mature infants who died at birth or shortly after. He found that some haemorrhages of the nerve fibre layer extended far out to the periphery, dislocating retinal elements and sometimes forming dense masses of blood.

He also claims to have seen capillary ruptures, a fact which must be doubted if one studies his technique: The fixed and stained retina was cut between blocks of cheese (!) after the fat had been extracted. This technique is bound to create artefacts and false conclusions, as indicated by Naumoff's opinion that the internal limiting membrane was easily penetrated by blood cells. In this respect the lithographs of Naumoff cannot be compared to the photographs obtained from epon-embedded material.

With or without knowledge of the microscopic details, the interpretation of the superficial haemorrhages as confined to the nerve fibre layer is almost always correctly given in the literature. The small extravasations are named linear or splinter-shaped. The medium ones are mainly called flame-shaped, sometimes fusiform, diamond-shaped or brush-strokes. Confluent haemorrhages do not really form a separate group, although some authors classify them as sheet-like (McKeown, 1941; Giles, 1960; Santamarina, 1969). Their appearance is also compared to that of a retinal thrombosis (Franceschetti and Balavoine, 1951; Yamanouchi, 1959; Brogi et al., 1962; Puskás and Szabó, 1961). The same seems to be meant by the expression of Jain and Gupta (1965): "Stormy sunset appearance".

Haemorrhages of the internal granular layer have already been described by Ulrich (1884) and Naumoff (1890). He also observed that the internal plexiform layer is a massive barrier difficult to pass for these haemorrhages. This type of haemorrhage is known from work with other diseases, e.g. venous thrombosis (Seitz, 1968). Duke-Elder (1967) calls them "dot and blot haemorrhages", arising from the capillary plexus of the exterior part of the internal granular layer. Their white centre could consist of fibrin coagula or masses of thrombocytes. This opinion is based on the classification of Foster Moore (1926), which could not be used for this presentation because of the impossibility in deciding whether the diamond-shaped or the rosette haemorrhage are those confined to the internal nuclear layer.

In connection with perinatal haemorrhages, this granular type is mentioned by Richman, but she believed that they were haemorrhages of the ganglion cell layer. Kauffman thought that they were possibly choroidal. If they were separated at all from other types, these haemorrhages seem to have been called: round, nummular or punctiform. Other names are "spongeous" (Paufique et al., 1965; Pannarale, 1966), "geographical" or "lake" haemorrhage (Baum and Bulpitt, 1970), "circular, comparable to a bunch of red flowers" (Tranou-Sphalangakou, 1968). They can be detected in the illustrations of Tranou-Sphalangakou (1968), Bulpitt and Baum (1969) and Wierhake (1971), but without clear descriptions. Baum and Bulpitt believed that they were situated under the internal limiting membrane.

In conclusion, it has to be said that the definition of the haemorrhages of the internal granular layer was either derived histologically without including ophthalmoscopic detail or, if the haermorrhages had been clearly seen clinically, their correlation with one of the retinal layers was nonetheless erroneus.

The hemispheric submembranacious haermorrhages have been compared to drops (Tranou-Sphalangakou, 1968), blobs (Baum and Bulpitt, 1970), little hats (Lomičková and Otradovec, 1956), vesicles (Moulene, 1956) and hills (Takeda, 1968). The brillant reflex on their summit has frequently been observed and is the best criterion as to whether this type of haemorrhage was properly defined as a separate group or not (Sidler-Huguenin, 1903; Wille, 1946; Belmonte-Gonzales, 1947; Grassi and Musini, 1950; Mayer and Maria, 1952; Tsópelas and Charamis, 1955; Motohashi and Kobayashi, 1960; Puskás and Szabó, 1961; Stefanini et al., 1968; Baum and Bulpitt, 1970). This superficial refléction was not always separated from the clot of fibrin in flat haemorrhages (Wille, 1946; Wierhake, 1971) though the two look very different.

A reflection of similar brightness on top of haemorrhages seems to occur only in children with haemorrhages related either to birth or to intracranial pressure. One explanation could be that the typical strong superficial reflection of the internal limiting membrane at this age is especially visible over the hemispheric haemorrhage. Another possibility is that the connection of Müller cells to the internal limiting membrane is especially close in children, the elevation thereby remaining restricted to a small and very prominent area, whereas in the adult large, flat elevations of the internal limiting membrane occur (Drews and Minckler, 1944).

The hemispheric submembranacious haemorrhages are hardly ever attributed to their proper location within the retina: Mayer and Maria (1952) call them preretinal or prechoroidal; Sorsby (1963), subretinal or choroidal; Coburn (1904) and Kauffman (1941) subhyaloidal. The most common expression is preretinal (Seissiger, 1929; Rico, 1939; Wille, 1946; Powelett and Townes, 1948; Baillard, 1953; Lemmingson and Stark, 1957; Yamanouchi, 1959; Motohashi and Kobayashi, 1960; Brogi et al., 1962; Paufique et al., 1965; Neuweiler and Onwudiwe, 1967; Stefanini et al., 1968; Tranou-Sphalangakou, 1968; Weiden, 1970). It was already suggested that this expression is not correct by Powelett and Townes (1948), who nevertheless continued to use it.

Only a few authors knew that these haemorrhages are situated under the internal limiting membrane (McKeown, 1941; Puskás and Szabó, 1961; Moulene, 1965; Duke-Elder, 1967). Some older publications, based on histological descriptions, ascribed them to their proper location. The same effusions with subarachnoidal haemorrhage in infants were also called preretinal (Sourdille, 1964; Hervouet, 1968), though the histology demonstrates an intact limiting membrane. This also applies to a study by Smith et al. (1957) with experimental retinal haemorrhages in the rhesus monkey.

The reason for the confusion is that no proper term existed. The specific cavity under the internal limiting membrane does not correspond to a retinoschisis. Therefore, the terms "subretinal", "intraretinal" and "subhyaloidal" from the CIBIS classification (1965) do not offer a proper designation. A new term, like "prenerval" or "sublaminar" could be difficult to understand. Therefore the author adopts the term "submembranacious" used by Fine and Yanoff (1972) in differentiating "subvitreal haemorrhage from sub-internal limiting membrane (i.e. superficial intraretinal)". This anatomically correct though still unusual expression "submembranacious" should be preferred to „preretinal", which is incorrect in this connection. The real preretinal, i.e. subhyaloidal and hyaloidal, haemorrhages will be discussed in this chapter, Sects. B.2 and B.3.

Reviewing the literature with correct knowledge of the ophthalmoscopic picture and the histologic correlation for the three types of intraretinal haemorrhages the author can find very few useful classifications. The most realistic classification seems to be that of Ciechanowska et al. (1974):

1. Flameshaped
2. Flat and round, light-red coloured
3. Thick and round, deep-red coloured, with reflection

Less valid are other recent classifications, as demonstrated by a few examples only:

Tranou-Sphalangakou (1968)

1. Linear or fusiform
2. Flame-shaped or circular
3. Preretinal, drop-like

Sezen (1970)

1. Flame-shaped, close to the disc
2. Light-red, irregular, superficial (explained as overlapping flame-shaped haemorrhages)
3. Round, deeplying, at the posterior pole

Wierhake (1971)

1. Nerve fibre layer, streak or flame-shaped, close to the disc, rarely with a white central spot
2. Oval, light-red, frequently with a central spot. mobile with the movement of the ophthalmoscope
3. Dark-red, between disc and macula, rarely with wandering central point
4. Macular haemorrhages corresponding to number 3
5. Haemorrhages comparable to central venous thrombosis

The most extreme example with seven different types was presented by Drozdowa (1951)

1. Flame-shaped and radial at the border of the disc
2. Patchy, with indistinct margins
3. Streaks, radial to the disc and along vessels
4. Brush-shaped
5. Circular with distinct margins
6. Splashes
7. Preretinal

Still, it is remarkable how seldom the optic phenomenon of the superficial reflex on hemispheric submembranacious haemorrhages has been distinguished from the white centre of the flat types of intraretinal haermorrhages.

B. Extraretinal Haemorrhages

The previous chapter dealt with haemorrhages originating in the superficial vasculated retinal layers and with their spread into all layers of the retina. Massive haemorrhages can extend to subretinal and preretinal spaces. Unfortunately the logic name "preretinal haemorrhage" should be avoided for this type because it has been so widely abused for bleeding retained by the internal limiting membrane, i.e. the submembranacious haemorrhages. They will be classified as subhyaloid and hyaloid according to their penetration through the hyaloid membrane although the penetration from the virtual subhyaloid space into the vitreous body seems to be the rule.

It must be discussed beforehand whether a subhyaloid space and a proper hyaloid membrane exist. According to electron-microscopic details, the vitreous structure is condensed into a cortical layer of about 100 μm (Rohen). Gärtner (1962, 1965) uses the term "vitreoretinal limiting layer" or "vitreo-retinaler Basalmembran-Fibrillenkomplex" to express that under physiologic conditions a unit is formed by vitreo-retinal adhesion. The splitting of this unit in the aging eye into a true internal limiting membrane of the retina and a hyaloid membrane is well known. That this splitting can occur in newborn infants as a fixation artefact is demonstrated by Fig. 20 (p. 23).

1. Subretinal Haemorrhages

Invasion of blood cells into the external nuclear layer has been demonstrated in Chap. III, Sect. A.2.b. Penetration of the external limiting membrane, forming true subretinal haemorrhages, has not been observed in this series. According to reliable literary reports they exist (Naumoff, 1890; von Hippel, 1898; Coburn, 1904; Drozdowa, 1951; Doege, 1969). These haemorrhages can only be derived from those of the inner nuclear layer, the deepest retinal layer containing capillaries.

The clinical aspect of perinatal subretinal haemorrhages seems not to have been observed; at least, there seem to be no precise descriptions.

2. Subhyaloid Haemorrhages

The invasion of blood cells into the virtual space between the hyaloid membrane and the internal limiting membrane of the retina is demonstrated in Fig. 49. A larger venule in the periphery is the source for this extravasation (Fig. 50). The blood cells have filled in the ganglion cell layer and the nerve fibre layer, the latter being rather flat in this peripheral area. From here, the internal limiting membrane become detached and finally burst. The penetrating blood cells split the hyaloid membrane from the internal limiting membrane, as can be studied in Fig. 51. The invasion of blood cells into the virtual subhyaloid space encounters the resistance of denser adhesions between the two membranes. Figure 52 demonstrates how, by such an adhesion, the mass of blood cells is subdivided into lenticular compartments. The hyaloid membrane seems to be ruptured at these adhesions, thereby allowing the blood cells to invade the vitreous body itself.

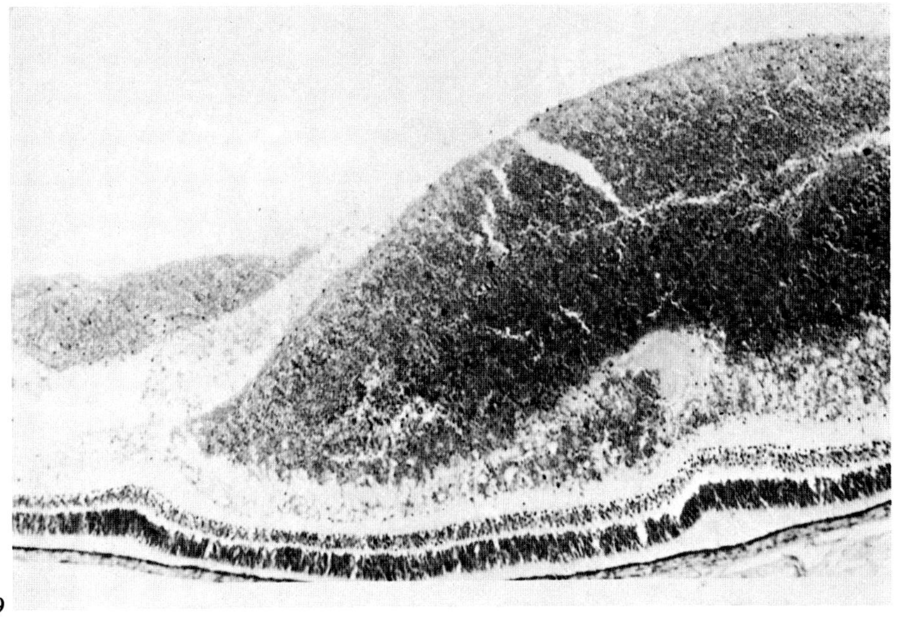

Figs. 49 and 50. Very extensive haemorrhage of retinal periphery. originating from larger venule with strong dilatation. Its rupture and fibrin thrombus demonstrated in detail in Fig. 50. Above this the submembranacious haemorrhage emerges. An additional pool of blood is visible over the internal limiting membrane and under the hyaloid membrane. Paraffin, haematoxilin-eosin. Fig. 49, x 100; Fig. 50, x 600

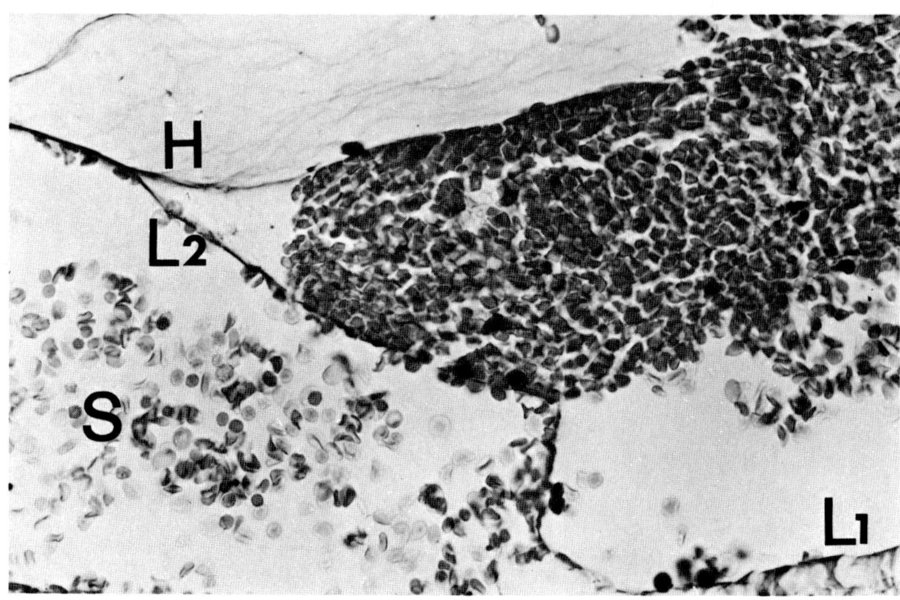

Fig. 51. Subhyaloid development of retinal haemorrhage. Intact vitreous body at *upper border.* Internal limiting membrane still in contact with Müller cells at *lower right corner* (L_1). Submembranacious haemorrhage (*S*) causes detachment of internal limiting membrane (L_2). At *upper left corner,* this membrane still in normal contact with hyaloid membrane (*H*). A cleavage of these two membranes is caused by subhyaloid haemorrhage progressing from *right border.* Rupture of internal limiting membrane, allowing this progression, not visible in this section. By shrinking of the vitreous body during fixation, the subhyaloid haemorrhage has been lifted from the internal limiting membrane. The submembranacious haemorrhage seems to be very loosely packed. Paraffin, PAS, x 500

3. Hyaloid (Vitreous) Haemorrhages

The further penetration of blood cells into the vitreous substance at a defect of the hyaloid membrane is demonstrated in Figure 53.

A gross section of partly fixed retina (Fig. 54) demonstrates an extensive subhyaloid haemorrhage hovering — the result of an artefact — over a submembranacious haemorrhage. On the level of the hyaloid membrane many ruptures have occurred and many invasions of blood cells are visible which appear shrub-shaped. Images like this gross section of Figures 52 and 53 must be looked upon as fortuitous "snap-shots" of a process. Once the internal limiting membrane is ruptured, the blood cells transcend the stage of subhyaloid haemorrhage and rapidly penetrate the gaps of the hyaloid membrane. Their penetration into the vitreous body rapidly decreases their visibility.

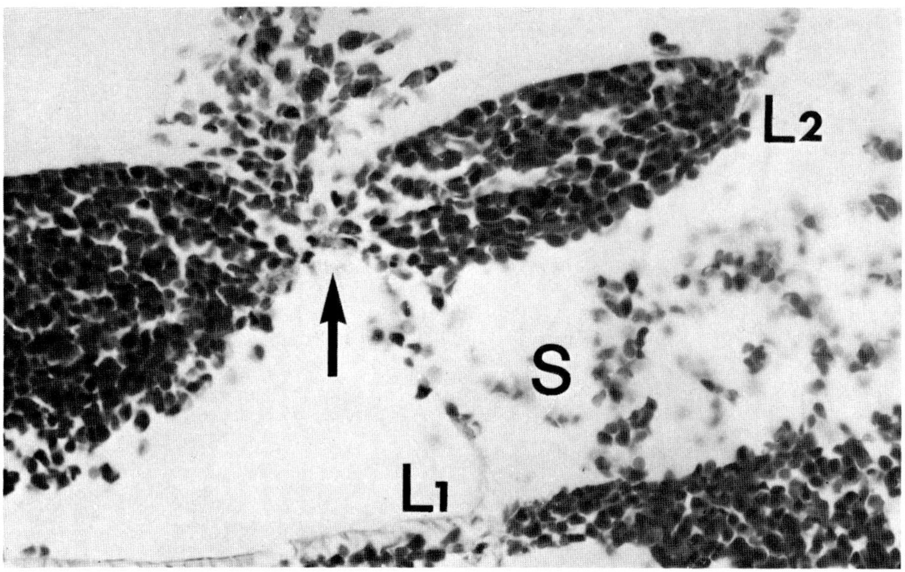

Fig. 52. Similar conditions to those in Fig. 51. Detachment of internal limiting membrane (L_1) from Müller cells at site of submembranacious haemorrhage (S). Artefactitious lifting of internal limiting membrane (L_2), causing loose packing of submembranacious haemorrhage (S). A close adhesion (*arrow*) of internal limiting membrane and hyaloid membrane causes rupture of latter and blood cells invade vitreous body. Paraffin, PTAH, x 500

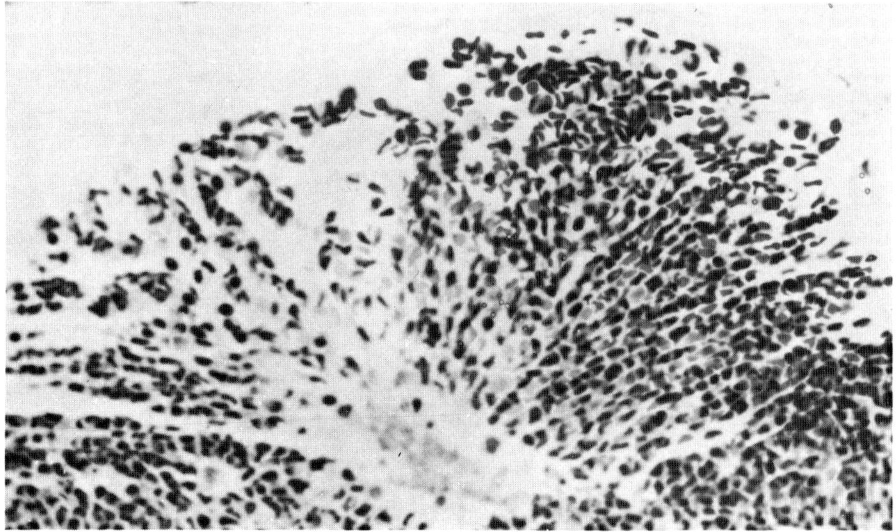

Fig. 53. Radial orientation of blood cells invading vitreous body from defect of hyaloid membrane. Epon after previous paraffin embedding, toluidine blue, x 500

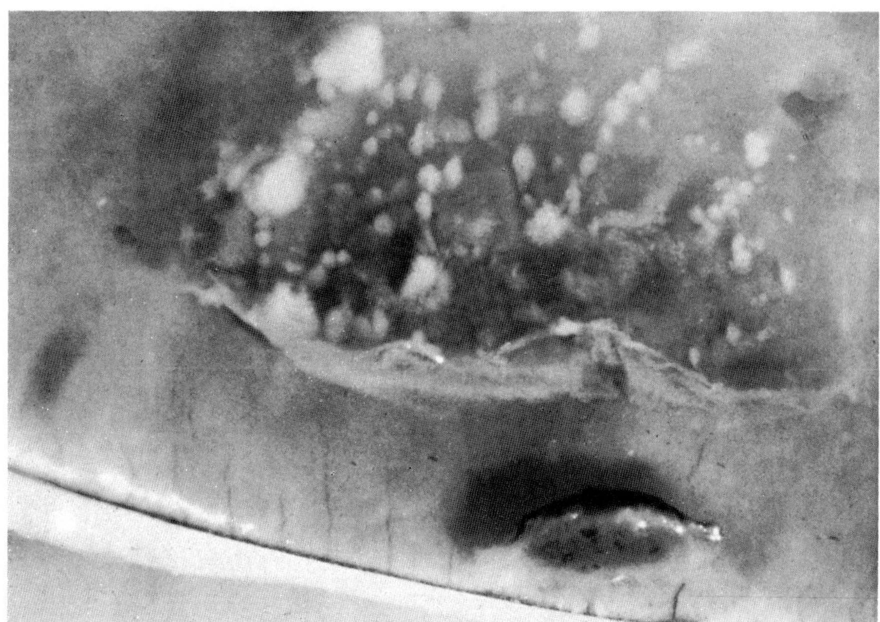

Fig. 54. Retina and vitreous body, fixation in formaldehyde. Section cuts through sub-membranacious haemorrhage, and above this hovers – as an artefact of fixation – an extensive subhyaloid haemorrhage. From surface, multiple tufts demonstrate invasion of blood cells into vitreous body, from multiple defects of hyaloid membrane

4. Discussion

In this clinical series several submembranacious haemorrhages were seen, all having a clear brillant reflection on their summit, indicating that the internal limiting membrane had not been penetrated.. In only one child, a true vitreous haemorrhage was seen, which had caused a diffuse blurring of the entire vitreous body a few hours after birth. After the rapid dissolution of this vitreous haemorrhage, a few days later, only a few indistinct relics of retinal haemorrhage were visible. The source of the vitreous haemorrhage could no longer be deduced.

There are reports about vitreous haemorrhage from histologic investigations: Coburn (1904) saw one case macroscopically and two cases in microscopic sections from 37 children. Lachmann (1927) found massive vitreous haemorrhages in the eyes of a child enucleated because of suspected glioma. He related the haemorrhage to obstetric trauma (forceps delivery). In addition, Eades' (1929) case of a stillborn infant with massive unilateral vitreous haemorrhage was seen in connection with obstetric trauma.

From the literature more clinical observations can be compiled. The definition of a vitreous haemorrhage is not always certain. Sometimes submemebranacious haemorrhages seem to be included (Duesberg and Tiburtius, 1958; Martinez and Grom, 1969). The following authors report on true vitreous or hyaloid haemorrhages:

Péhu and Bonamour (1938): 483 children, two cases of vitreous haemorrhage

McKeown (1941): 498 children, three vitreous haemorrhages, one of them (after a forceps delivery) so massive that fundus details were indistinct

Nevinny-Stickel (1954): 159 children, six vitreous haemorrhages, two of which were still visible after 7 days

Pannarale (1966): 550 children, one vitreous haemorrhage

Nehrdich (1968): One heavy child asphyctic, massive vitreous haemorrhages, still visible after 8 weeks; one child after vacuum extraction, with vitreous haemorhage, still visible after 3 weeks

Panagiotou et al. (1968): 1220 children, one vitreous haemorrhage

Martinez and Grom (1969): 122 children, six vitreous haemorrhages (?)

Richter (1969): 1145 children, one vitreous haemorrhage

Taleb Bendiab (1972): 100 children, one vitreous haemorrhage

A special type of vitreous haemorrhage seems to occur in immature infants.

Naunton and Forrester (1955): Vitreous opacity and congested vessels at the 9th day, bilateral vitreous haemorrhage at the 12th day resulting in strabism after 8 months

Braendstrup (1969): Five of the children with vitreous haemorrhages were immature

Fontaine (1971): Three immature children with massive vitreous haemorrhage.

Wiznia and Price (1976): Three immature infants with respiratory distress syndrome and vitreous haemorrhages, presumably caused by a mild form of disseminated intravascular coagulation

We can add an original observation of an immature child presenting bilateral massive vitreous haemorrhage at the age of 6 weeks after oxygen therapy. After the clearing up of the vitreous body the retina was normal. These cases have no relation to true retinopathy of prematurity and no connection with intracranial haemorrhages. They are not yet present at birth and must have a different cause than perinatal haemorrhages.

C. White Fibrin Thrombi of Vessel Ruptures and Fibrin Emboli in Retinal Vessels

The white thrombi occluding vessel ruptures have already been cited in discussing the sources of different types of haemorrhage. The material of these fibrin coagula and the possible relation to fibrin emboli will now be discussed. White centres of retinal haemorrhages of different origin have been described as Roth's spots (Kennedy and Wise, 1965; Wise et al., 1971). Of these only the ones found in aplastic anaemia have been proven to consist of fibrin.

There have been many speculations about the nature of the white centre of perinatal retinal haemorrhages. The wandering reflex on submembranacious haemorrhages has not always been separated from the immobile white mass in flat haemorrhages. Wille (1949) writes about flame-shaped haemorrhages with a central "reflex", Koyama (1959) about flame-shaped haemorrhages with and without a "vacuole". Richman

(1937) tries to explain the centre as serum, François and Tranos (1975) discuss it as an aggregation of leucocytes. The aspect of the white centre as such is well documented, though not explained with the illustrations of Wille (1946), Tranou-Sphalangakou (1968), Baum and Bulpitt (1970) and Wierhake (1971). It seems not to be presented on fundus paintings. The illustrations by Richman (1937b) seem to suffer especially from the late observation date.

The original illustrations here prove that the white centre is practically a constant feature. Only sources of bleeding in the ganglion cell layer can be hidden under the further spread of the haemorrhage in the nerve fibre layer, Submembranacious haemorrhages may disclose their fibrin thrombus, but only if the thrombus is situated very far in their periphery.

Elelctron-microscopic studies have been conducted to investigate the material of the white coagulum (Fig. 55). The important thrombus of the inset (cf. Fig. 20) was studied, and the same fibrillar material was found within the lumen of the vessel and outside the rupture. This material linked in the typical way blood cells with platelets within the vessel and invaded the spaces between the Müller cells. The electron-microscopic appearance corresponds to fibrin fibrillae. With PTAH staining there was a positive reaction. Therefore it seems reasonable to interprete the white coagulum as a fibrin thrombus.

Frequently the thrombus itself is surrounded by a halo containing fewer blood cells than the surrounding haemorrhagic area. The simplest explanation seems to be that these gaps had originally been filled with loosely packed fibrin, which then contracted, leaving serum in the space (cf. Figs. 10, 20, 29, 37).

Thus the connection between retinal haemorrhages and fibrin thrombi is explained. It remains to be discussed whether intravasal fibrin emboli could also have a relation to these haemorrhages. Immature infants suffering from intrauterine and sometimes perinatal asphyxia can develop intravasal coagulation, with fibrin emboli visible in histologic sections (Bleyl and Büsing, 1970). These emboli have not yet been described in the retina but seem to have been seen in ciliary veins by de Groot and Friedenwald (1957).

In the numerous complete serial sections prepared for this work, many intravasal fibrin emboli were visible within the retina. Figure 56 demonstrates a small embolus filling a small retinal arteriole. Missing incorporated blood cells or aggregations of platelets indicate that embolus formation occurred prior to death. A larger intravenous embolus is seen in Fig. 57. Here also a haemorrhage of the internal nuclear layer is present, with a small fibrin thrombus occluding the capillary rupture. As in all other serial sections (cf. Plate XII), no relation between intravasal fibrin emboli and retinal haemorrhages was detectable. Although both occur mainly in the perinatal period, they occur in different groups of children. Retinal haemorrhages and their fibrin thrombi are more frequently found in mature than in immature infants (cf. Chap. VII, Sect. C.4). Intravasal fibrin emboli tend to occur with immature infants with a birth weight under 1000 g and a hypercoagulability caused by asphyxia leading to a consumtion of coagulative factors. The resulting intravasal coagulation must be expected with moribund infants. These do not appear to have beem examined, so that the ophthalmoscopic appearance of these emboli, if visible at all, is unknown. The funduscopy of healthy mature children for the study of perinatal haemorrhages certainly does not reveal intravasal fibrin emboli.

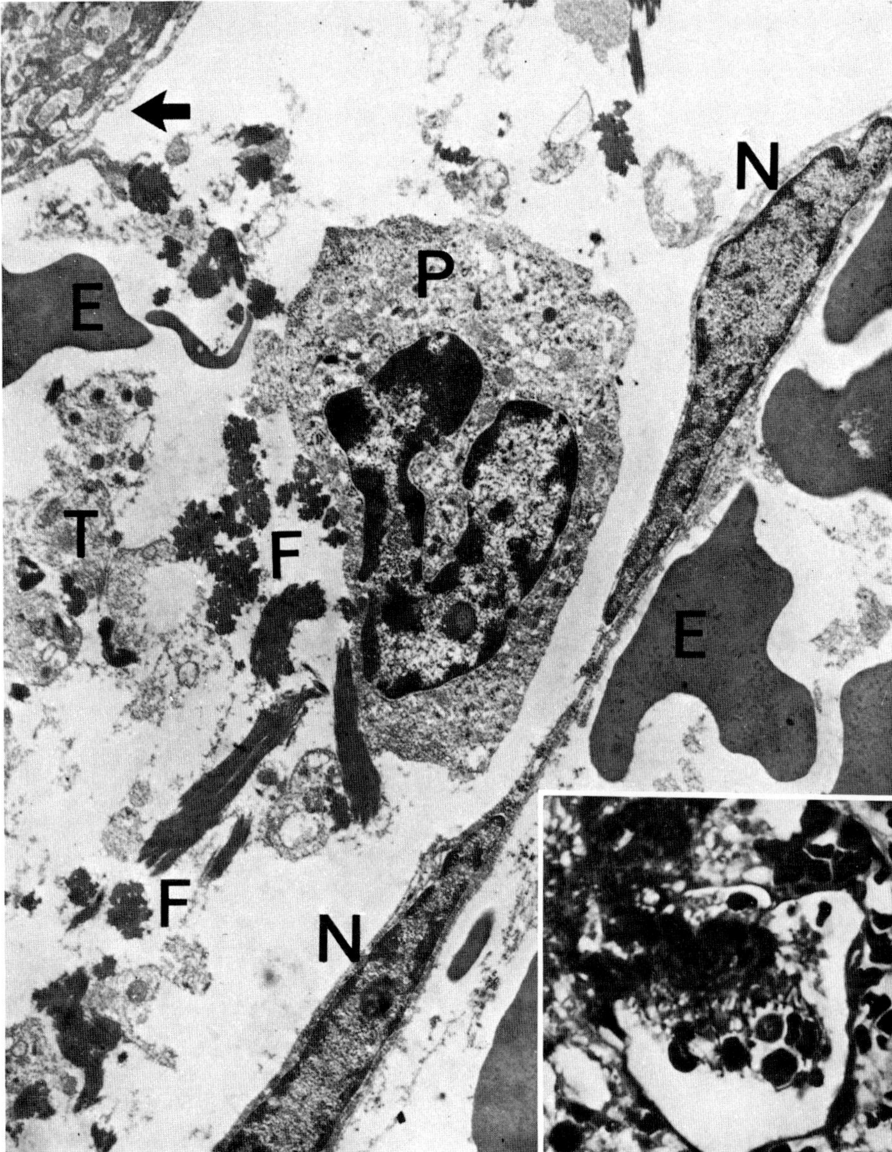

Fig. 55. Electron-microscopic details of venular wall close to vessel rupture demonstrated in *inset* (cf. Fig. 20). Section corresponds to right lower border of venular wall. *N,* nuclei of endothelial cells; *E,* erythrocytes within tissue (*right side*) and vessel lumen (*left side*); *P,* polymorphonuclear leucocyte; *T,* thrombocytes; *F,* meshwork of fine fibrils interpreted as fibrin, connecting cellular elements to thrombus (*arrow*) composed of same material, reembedded in epon, x 10,000

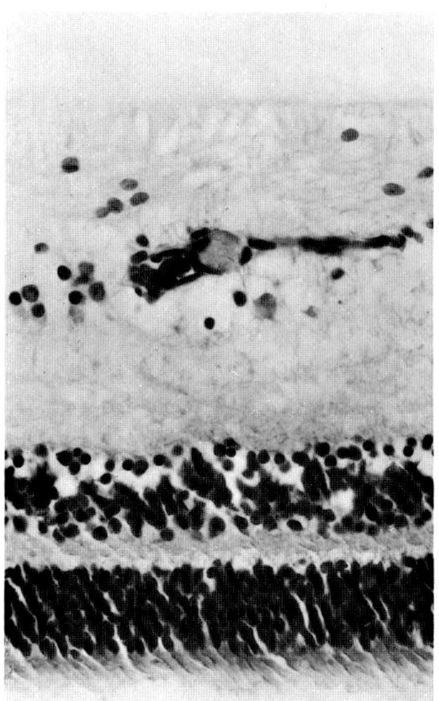

Fig. 56. Fibrin embolus of intravital origin in retinal arteriole. No haemorrhage in vicinity. Paraffin, Goldner, x 500

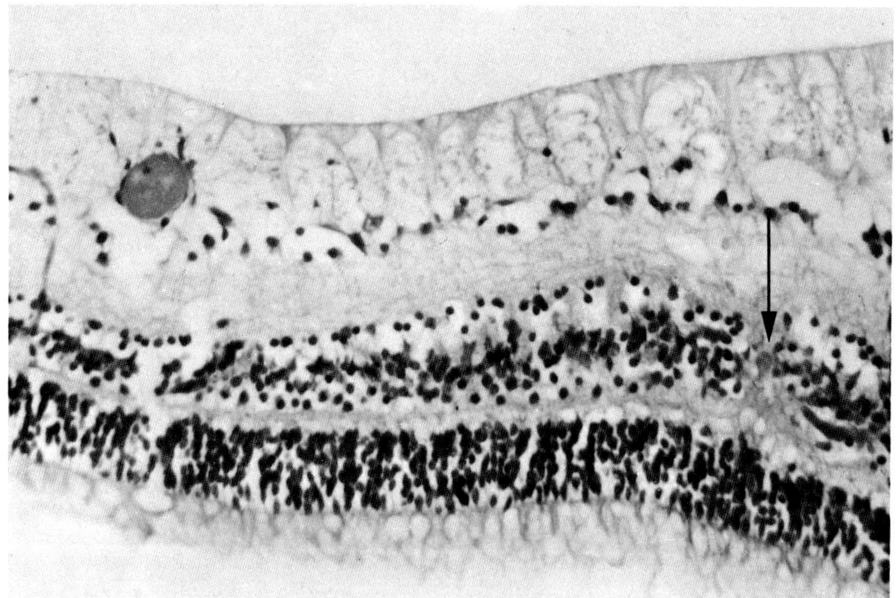

Fig. 57. Retinal venule, entirely occluded by fibrin embolus of intravital origin. No reaction in surrounding tissues. Haemorrhage of internal granular layer originates from capillary rupture (*arrow*). Cellular elements pushed aside in centre

Besides the undoubted existence of retinal haermorrhages caused by rhexis, dia-pedesis has been discussed as a cause (Montalcini, 1897; Jirman, 1947; Grigera, 1964; Planten and v.d. Schaaf, 1971). Certainly it would be difficult to prove that diapedesis does not occur but, from our material, it was impossible to demonstrate that it does. In complete serial sections, all haemorrhages yielded a source of bleeding, even when a capillary was involved. Single blood cells within the tissue were not encountered. The fundus photographs, in addition, only demonstrate haemorrhages that are explained by vessel ruptures.

It is still astonishing that such a simple item as a clearly visible white centre at the site of a vessel rupture was overlooked by so many investigators and, when it was seen by others, the simple explanation of a fibrin thrombus was never proposed. Once more ophthalmology offers the possibility of observing by direct in vivo examination another generally interesting aspect of vessel pathology.

D. Summary

According to their location in different retinal layers, the perinatal haemorrhages can be subdivided into several intraretinal and extraretinal groups. A valuable classification can only be obtained by a synopsis of in vivo examinations, including fundus photo-graphs, with photography of post mortem retinae and complete serial sections. The resulting classification is the following:

A. Intraretinal Haemorrhages. From the rupture of a capillary or venule in the nerve fibre layer or ganglion cell layer, or from a capillary rupture within the internal nuclear layer, the extravasations spread within their own layer or penetrate other layers, still leaving the internal and the external limiting membranes intact.

1. Flame-Shaped Haemorrhages of the Nerve Fibre Layer. The most frequent type of haemorrhages, originating from the ganglion cell layer or from the nerve fibre layer itself and always shaped according to the orientation of the fibres. According to the size of the vessel ruptured, they are linear, fusiform, flame-shaped or confluent. In most cases a white fibrin thrombus occluding the vessel rupture indicates their centre. This can be hidden in a haemorrhage from the ganglion cell layer.

2. Granular Haemorrhages of the Internal Granular Layer. According to the vas-cularization of the internal granular layer with rather uniform capillaries, these haem-morrhages are less frequent and more uniform in their spread. Usually confined to the internal granular layer, their borderline has a dendritic or granular appearance, shaped by the arrangement of blood cells in small vertical columns between the cellular ele-ments. The capillary rupture is occluded by a fibrin thrombus, also ophthalmoscop-ically visible as the white centre of this haemorrhage. Penetration into the external granular layer is frequent. An eruption through the very dense barrier of the internal plexiform layer seems to be a rare exception.

3. Hemispheric Submembranacious Haemorrhages. This characteristic develop-ment of the haemorrhages can occur close to the macular area or in the periphery, where the nerve fibre layer is flat and offers few possibilities for spread. Here the

Müller cells become stretched, and finally their connection with the internal limiting membrane will be torn. The extravasation then dislocates the detached internal limiting membrane, causing the ophthalmoscopically visible brillant light reflex on the summit of the protuberance. Still confined to retinal tissue, this haemorrhage should not be called "preretinal", as the term is misleading. If involved, the fovea centralis can be reached by this submembranacious spread.

B. Extraretinal Haemorrhages.

1. Subretinal Haemorrhages. Penetration of the external limiting membrane exists according to reliable reports. It was not found in this series.

2. Subhyaloid Haemorrhages. Penetrating the very resistant internal limiting membrane, a submembranacious haemorrhage can extend into the virtual space between hyaloid membrane and internal limiting membrane. The term "preretinal haemorrhage" is avoided because it has been abused for submembranacious haemorrhages. Subhyaloid haemorrhages seem to represent just a step towards the development of the next type.

3. Hyaloid Haemorrhages. After having entered the virtual subhayloid space, blood cells will enter the vitreous body itself through numerous defects of the hyaloid membrane. These are caused by closer junctions with the internal limiting membrane. These true vitreous haemorrhages are rare complications of perinatal haemorrhages.

The Fibrin Thrombus of Retinal Haemorrhages. In the majority of flat haemorrhages the centre is indicated by a white spot. This consists of a thrombus of fibrin occluding the vessel rupture, with an intravasal and extravasal part. The simple explanation of this white centre as fibrin was not found in the literature.

Zusammenfassung

Entsprechend ihrer Lage in verschiedenen Netzhautschichten werden die perinatalen Blutungen in intraretinale und extraretinale Gruppen eingeteilt. Eine Klassifikation von Wert kann nur durch eine synoptische Analyse der Lebendbeobachtungen, Fundusfotografien im Vergleich mit Retinafotografien und Serienschnitten verstorbener Kinder erzielt werden. Die sich ergebende Klassifizierung ist die folgende:

A. Intraretinale Blutungen. Aus einer Kapillar- oder Venolen-Ruptur in der Nervenfaserschicht oder Ganglienzellschicht oder auch einer Kapillar-Ruptur in der inneren Körnerschicht kann eine Blutung sich in der eigenen oder angrenzenden Schichten ausbreiten, während noch die Lamina limitans interna und externa intakt sind.

1. Die flammenförmigen Blutungen der Nervenfaserschicht. Der häufigste Blutungstyp mit Blutungsquelle in der Nervenfaserschicht oder in der Ganglienzellschicht ist in der Begrenzung immer durch die Nervenfaserschicht geformt. Je nach der Größe des rupturierten Gefäßes treten sie als strichförmige, spindelförmige, flammenförmige oder aus mehreren Quellen konfluierende Blutungen auf. Meist wird ihr Zentrum markiert von einem weißen Fibrinthrombus, der die Gefäßruptur verschließt. Bei Blutungen der Ganglienzellschicht kann dieser Thrombus verborgen sein.

2. Die granulären Blutungen der inneren Körnerschicht. Entsprechend der Versorgung der inneren Körnerschicht mit ziemlich gleichmäßigen Kapillaren sind auch die Blutungen ziemlich einheitlich in ihrer Ausdehnung und weniger häufig. Ihre granuläre oder dendritische Begrenzung ergibt sich durch das Arrangement der Blutzellen in kleinen senkrechten Säulen zwischen den Zellen der inneren Körnerschicht. Auch hier ist die Kapillar-Ruptur durch einen Fibrinthrombus markiert, der als weißes Zentrum sichtbar wird. Ein Vordringen in die äußere Körnerschicht ist häufig, eine Eruption durch die sehr dichte Barriere der inneren plexiformen Schicht scheint eine seltene Ausnahme zu sein.

3. Die halbkugeligen submembranösen Blutungen. Eine charakteristische Ausdehnung der Oberflächenblutungen kann in der Maculagegend oder in der Peripherie auftreten, wo die geringe Mächtigkeit der Nervenfaserschicht kaum Möglichkeiten zur Expansion bietet. Hier werden die Müllerschen Zellen überdehnt und schließlich ihre Fußplatten von der Lamina limitans interna abgerissen. Diese wird durch das Extravasat abgehoben und vorgewölbt, wobei der ophthalmoskopisch sichtbare brillante Oberflächenreflex über der Blutung entsteht. Da sie noch auf retinales Gewebe begrenzt bleiben, ist die Bezeichnung „praeretinal" irreführend. Wenn die avaskuläre Fovea betroffen ist, kann sie nur durch diese Blutungsform invadiert sein.

B. Extraretinale Blutungen.

1. Subretinale Blutungen. Penetration der Lamina limitans externa wurde in der eigenen Serie nicht beobachtet, kommt jedoch nach verläßlichen Literaturangaben vor.

2. Die subhyaloidalen Blutungen. Durch Penetration der sehr widerstandsfähigen Lamina limitans interna kann eine submembranöse Blutung sich in den virtuellen Spaltraum zwischem Membrana hyaloidea und Membrana limitans interna ausdehnen. Der Ausdruck „praeretinal" wird hier vermieden, weil er für submembranöse Blutungen mißbraucht wurde. Die subhyaloidalen Blutungen scheinen nur einen vorübergehenden Schritt darzustellen, auf dem Wege zum nächsten Typ:

3. Die hyaloidalen Blutungen. Nach Eindringen in den virtuellen subhyaloidalen Spaltraum dringen die Blutzellen schnell in den Glaskörper vor, und zwar an den Defekten der Membrane hyaloidea, die durch das Ausreißen dichterer Verbindungen mit der Lamina limitans interna entstehen. Diese echten Glaskörperblutungen sind seltene Komplikationen perinataler Blutungen.

Der Fibrinthrombus retinaler Blutungen. In der Mehrzahl der Flächenblutungen wird das Zentrum durch einen weißen Fleck markiert. Dieser besteht aus einem Fibrinthrombus, der die Gefäßruptur verschließt und einen intravasalen und einen extravasalen Anteil hat. Die sehr einfache Erklärung des weißen Blutungszentrums als Fibrin ist merkwürdigerweise in der Literatur nicht beschrieben worden.

IV. Location

A. Clinical Reports

Early investigators (Schleich, 1884; von Sicherer, 1907; Juler, 1926) emphasized that if the retina is affected by haemorrhages this occurs mainly at the posterior pole, in the area of the disc and macula or along the main vessels. The attached plates, particularly in more extensive retinal haemorrhages, clearly demonstrate this preference for the posterior pole. Even with sufficient pupil dilatation and with the use of an indirect ophthalmoscope, few haemorrhages were seen in the periphery or the equatorial area. Plate II illustrates a fundus unusual in this respect: a few haemorrhages in the centre and a single submembranacious haemorrhage far outside the central fundus. This proves that peripheral location is not necessarily linked with massive haemorrhages, as some authors claimed (Mayer and Maria, 1952; Tsópelas and Charamis, 1955; Maertens and Götz, 1967). However, one will certainly find the periphery more frequently affected with multiple haemorrhages in severe cases.

Like the extravasations in adults with central vein occlusion, the concentration of haemorrhages at the posterior pole is explained by the dense vascularization in this area. Whether these capillaries are really arranged in separate layers is a matter for discussion (Podestà and Ullerich, 1956; Toussaint et al., 1961; Lieb and Bielefeld, 1967; Rohen, 1969). It is at least certain that vessels piercing the internal plexiform layer almost vertically feed a loose meshwork of capillaries of the internal granular layer. From the periphery to the centre the capillaries are more densely arranged, and their stratification is higher within the nerve fibre layer and the ganglion cell layer. An additional dense network of vessels surrounds the disc (Duke-Elder, 1961). Thus the close arrangement of venules and capillaries at the posterior pole easily explains the higher incidence of vessel ruptures in this area.

B. Histology

Contrary to clinical observation in post mortem retinae, haemorrhages are frequently seen far outside the centre, up to the ora serrata. This also applies to the eyes, the central fundi of which are presented in Plates X and XI. Both had several haemorrhages at the equatorial and oral periphery. Figure 58 illustrates a flat haemorrhage of the nerve fibre layer with spread in perivascular spaces and in close relation to the ora serrata. Not only flat haemorrhages have been found in the periphery but also submembranacious haemorrhages.

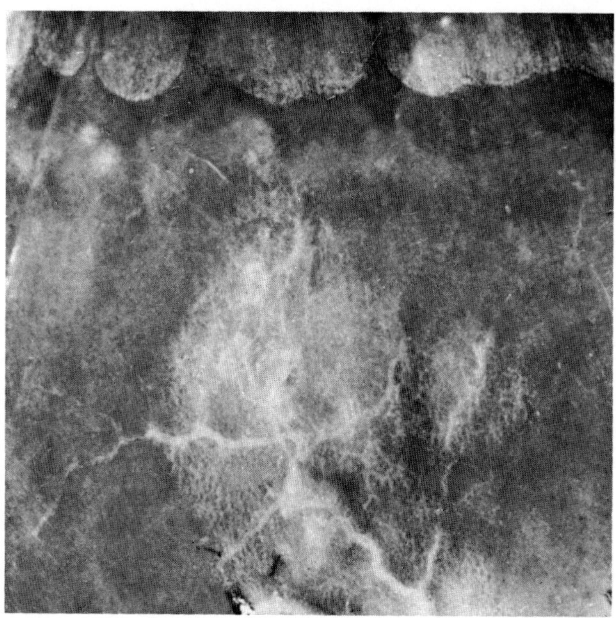

Abb. 58. Peripheral retina after fixation in formaldehyde. Blood cells brownish-white. Relation to ora serrata visible. A frequent finding in post mortem specimens

The few communications based on histologic examinations confirm the frequent affection of the peripheral retina, including the ora serrata (Ulrich, 1884; von Hippel, 1898: mainly in the oral periphery; Coburn, 1904: more peripheral than reported by the other — i.e. the clinical — investigators; Jacobs, 1928: no predilection for a certain retinal region; Reese et al., 1952: 10% oral affection in immature infants; Yoshioka, 1954: oral affection in immature infants).

There seems to be a definite difference between two groups, i.e. the healthy children seen under clinical examination on the one hand and the children dying after birth — some of them immature — on the other. With immature children, the not yet fully differentiated retinal periphery and its vessels might possibly be more inclined to haemorrhage. But certainly not only immature infants have peripheral retinal haemorrhages. Jacobs differentiated between the two groups: 7 out of 8 mature newborns had haemorrhages. In Naumoff's interesting series there were 22 immature infants without retinal haemorrhages and 12 mature infants with a birth weight between 2950 und 4550 g with haemorrhages in the central and peripheral retina.

While the author was aware of the possibility of peripheral retinal haemorrhage, he was unable to find more than a few examples of this in clinical observation. This is probably due partly to the difficulties of examination and partly to the fact that these haemorrhages occur less frequently in healthy children.

C. Macular Haemorrhage

The macular localization of retinal haemorrhages is of special interest because of its possible relation to amblyopia. Only in submembranacious haemorrhages can the fovea be involved. From the vascularized surrounding area a haemorrhage can invade the avascular centre by detaching the internal limiting membrane.

Histologically however, other affections have also been described: Naumoff (1890) saw the penetration of macular haemorrhages into the subretinal and the pre-retinal space. Von Hippel (1898) published the photograph of a massive subretinal haemorrhage which had penetrated the external limiting membrane in the macular area. Besides that, he found a submembranacious haemorrhage in the equatorial region, penetrating the internal limiting membrane. The similarity of the periphery to the macular area has been discussed. It is due to the thin layer of nerve fibres providing little space for the extension of the haemorrhage. Once the internal limiting membrane is detached, its further elevation from the Müller cells will develop in a centrifugal direction, as Plates I, VII and IX demonstrate. Here the eccentric origin of the haemorrhage is visible, as is its progression towards the fovea. It seems as if the internal limiting membrane is more easily detached in the foveal area than in surrounding areas.

In this work macular or foveal affection have been carefully noted. Among the 200 children serving as a control group of "normal cases" 78 were found with retinal haemorrhage, among which 8 had foveal affection (bilateral in one case).

In the case of 12 other children, the surface reflex of the macula was touched by a haemorrhage. These relations differ in groups with a higher incidence of haemorrhage. Thus, among 26 children after vacuum extraction there were 19 with haemorrhages, 7 with foveal involvement (bilateral in 2 of them) and 7 with affection of the macular area.

Exact figures on foveal involvement are unfortunately hard to obtain from the literature. In most cases the incidence of any retinal haemorrhage whatsoever is the only datum given. If central affection is mentioned, it is still impossible to determine whether it was really the fovea that was affected.

In 1900 Paul reported on macular affection: Among 200 children there were 17 bilateral and 10 unilateral cases with macular involvement mainly at the border. Figures on foveal involvement are lacking. Table 1 is an attempt to summarize the references. Unusual among these references is the report by Jochmus (1968), who found macular haemorrhages in 3/4 of the cases with haemorrhages. Possibly at the late examination date (up to the 1st week), smaller haemorrhages had already resorbed and only submembranacious haemorrhages of the centre remained. There are no other reports about a tendency for macular haemorrhage to develop in immature infants.

Table 1. Incidence of macular haemorrhages

Author	Year	Total series	Retinal haem.	Macular haem.	Remarks
Paul	1900	200	69	27	Macular area
Sykes	1931	312	74	13	
Croci and Scardaccione	1940	1000	292	90	
Powelett and Townes	1948	250	26	2	
Drozdova	1951	638	127	60	Macular area
Koyama	1959	409	105	3	Spontaneous delivery
		71	27	9	Forceps delivery
Yohitda et al.	1961	510	133	14	(14 eyes, 133 cases)
Pannarale	1966	550	143	48	Macular area
Birich and Peretitskaja	1968	1120	280	8	(8 eyes) extended macular haemorrh.
Franceschetti	1968	?	20%–25%	4%	
Fung et al.	1968	1000	264	43	6 bilateral
Jochmus	1968	451	56	3/4 of cases	Premature infants only
Doege	1969	1205	289	147	
von Barsewisch	1972	200	78	8	Spontaneous deliveries
		26	19	7	Vacuum extractions
Taleb Bendiab	1972	100	29	6	
von Noorden and Khodadoust	1973	1000	245	18	
Ciechanowski et al.	1974	232	55	26	Close to fovea

D. Bilaterality

In this author's series of 200 normal children with 78 retinal haemorrhages there were 43 bilateral and 35 unilateral cases. In the other group with more haemorrhages after vacuum extraction, the prevalence of bilateral involvement is more significant: 14 bilateral cases as compared to 5 unilateral cases.

From the literature no uniform opinion can be derived. Possibly the cause lies in the heterogeneity of the groups, although it seems more likely that each series is too small for statistical evaluation. Even if most authors find a higher incidence of bilateral involvement, an investigation so thoroughly done as that of Wierhake, with fundus photographs of all cases, comes to a result contradicting those of most other authors: She found a slight prevalence of unilateral haemorrhages.

The results compiled from the literature are to be found in Table 2.

Table 2. Bilaterality of retinal haemorrhages

Author	Year	Bilateral	Unilateral
Sykes	1931	39	35
Tadashi and Fujimori	1941	5	3
Vancea	1941	18	11
Wille	1946	113	139
Cook and Glascock	1951	16	16
Drozdova	1951	76	51
Cavrot	1956	35	49
Konstantopais	1956	24	22
Lomikova and Otradovec	1956	58%	41%
Crehange	1958	20	14
Duesberg and Tiburtius	1958	54%	46%
Casanovas et al.	1959	94	80
Mao	1959	67%	33%
Mijares	1959	2	22
Yamanouchi	1959	12	5
Motohashi and Kobayashi	1960	22	21
Yohita et al.	1961	66	67
Brogi et al.	1962	89	58
Kawakami et al.	1963	44	48
Moulene	1965	50	16
Pannarale	1966	107	36
Neuweiler and Onwudiwe	1967	217	140
Sachsenweger	1967	61%	39%
Bachmann et al.	1968	44	59 [a]
Takeda	1968	63	78
Lukaszewicz and Zaporowski	1969	4	26
Wierhake	1971	57	60
Barsewisch	1972	43	35 [a]
		14	5 [b]
Pommer	1972	50	46
Taleb Bendiab	1972	16	13
Ciechanowski et al.	1974	14	41

a   Occipital presentation.
b   Vacuum extraction.

E. Summary

All types of perinatal retinal haemorrhages are more frequently encountered at the posterior pole. Haemorrhages in the periphery seem to be either rare in mature infants or are frequently overlooked in clinical examinations. In histologic series, which in many cases include immature infants. peripheral haemorrhages including the oral periphery are frequently found.

Concerning the discussion of amblyopia due to retinal haemorrhages, only macular involvement can be of importance. Unfortunately literary reports are seldom precise about a true foveal location. These central haermorrhages can only belong to the type of submembranacious extravasation, originating from vessel ruptures close to the macula and detaching the central internal limiting membrane.

Perinatal haemorrhages seem to occur more frequently bilaterally than unilaterally.

Zusammenfassung

Alle Typen der perinatalen Netzhautblutungen finden sich häufiger im hinteren Pol mit seiner dichteren Vaskularisation. Periphere Blutungen scheinen bei reifen Kindern teils übersehen zu werden, teils wirklich selten vorzukommen. In histologischen Serien, die teilweise viele Frühgeborene umfassen, sind periphere Blutungen bis zur Oragegend häufig.

Bezüglich der diskutierten Amblyopieentstehung sind von den Retinablutungen nur die der Macula von Bedeutung. Unglücklicherweise sind aber die Literaturangaben höchst ungenau über eine wirklich foveale Beteiligung. Diese zentralen Blutungen können nur in der Form der submembranösen Kugelblutungen auftreten, die von Gefäßrupturen in der Maculaumgebung ausgehen und die Lamina limitans interna zentripetal abheben.

Perinatale Netzhautblutungen scheinen häufiger bilateral als unilateral vorzukommen.

V. Clinical Course

A. Onset

Königstein believed the haemorrhages to begin after birth with the arteriolization of blood. Three years later Schleich (1884) assumed that the bleeding occurrred during delivery due to deformation of the head. This opinion was confirmed by Naumoff's examinations of children who died during birth and has not been doubted since. It is also interesting to note that haemorrhages are observed after ceasarian section, but mainly after an attempted labour.

Mayer and Maria (1952) and Grigera (1964) tried to analyse the onset of perinatal haemorrhages by injecting the mother with fluorescein, prior to delivery or during the first stage of labour (Grigera). They found the infantile haemorrhages not to be fluorescent, and believed this proved the haemorrhages had occurred during the second stage. Since the appearance of fluorescein-positive haemorrhages is not described, the whole calculation seems to contain too many unknown facts.

B. Resorption

The haemorrhages present after birth dissolve rapidly, with few exceptions, as has been confirmed by all investigators since Königstein (1881). The finest linear haemorrhages can disappear within 24 h.

In this connection the very thorough study of Giles (1960) is of special interest. He examined 100 children 1 h after delivery and found 40 affected with haemorrhages. Reexamination of the same children on the next day showed that only 36 still had haemorrhages, i.e. in 1/10 of the cases the extravasation was resorbed. On the third day only 25% and on the fourth only 20% of the haemorrhages were found. Corresponding to the quick dissolution of haemorrhages demonstrated upon reexamination is the decrease of visible haemorrhage with advancing examination dates. Table 3 gives the references for this dependence. In this series only some special cases were reexamined, since the quick resorption of haemorrhages in general is well known (Belmonte-Gonzales, 1947; Drozdowa, 1951; Pentini, 1951; Petrowa, 1956; Jain and Gupta, 1965).

Ishikawa (1959) reports on the mean time of resorption: light haemorrhages, 3.6 days, medium haemorrhages, 5.2 days and severe haemorrhages, 8.8 days. Koyama (1959) reexamined 111 children and found the haemorrhages entirely dissolved by the 7th day for 85 children, by the 14th day for 18, by the 30th day for 5, by the 60th day for 2 and by the 90th day for 2. Pannarale's figures (1966) are similar: By the 7th and

Table 3. Dependence of incidence of retinal haemorrhages on the examination date (cases with haemorrhages/cases examined = percentage)

Author and year	1st day of life	2nd	3rd	4th	5th	6th	7th	8th	9th
Schleich, 1884	$<$ 4 h $<$12 h up to 2nd day	50% 32% 26.5%	After the 2nd day 15%						
Chase et al., 1950	2/ 25 = 8%	4/119 = 3.4%	9/186 = 4.8%	1/125 = 0.8%	2/145 = 1.3%	2/120 = 1.7%	2/96 = 2.1%	0/18	0/5
Dolcet and Ferrer, 1954	10/ 52 = 19.2%	12/ 50 = 24%	7/ 36 = 19.4%	2/ 26 = 7.7%	0/ 35	1/ 14 = 7.1%	0/ 7		
Yamanouchi, 1959	10/ 31	4/ 17	1/ 10	1/ 8	1/ 5	0/ 7			
Giles, 1960 [a]	49/199 = 40%	36%	25%	20%					
Jain and Gupta, 1965	$<$ 6 h 40.7% $<$12 h 28.6% $<$24 h 24.6%	5/ 21 = 23.2%	1/ 19 = 11.1%						
Paufique et al., 1965	38/111 = 34.8%			24%	10.5%				
Krebs and Jäger, 1966	25%	16%	ca. 15%	9–10%					
Bachmann et al., 1968 [b]	35/ 62	9/ 21	6/ 13	3/ 10	2/ 4				
Stefanini et al., 1968	10/ 52 = 19% [c] 22/ 46 = 38% [b]			8/ 52 = 15% 16/ 46 = 35%					
Sezen, 1970	?/709 = 18.9%	?/304 = 12.5%	?/225 = 2.6%						
Tranou-Sphalangakou, 1968	34/109 = 31.4%	13/ 43 = 30%	9/ 37 = 24.3%						
Baum and Bulpitt, 1970	20/100 = 20% within 12 h 16/ 39 = 31%	6/ 52 = 11.5%	7/ 57 = 12%		Mainly premature infants				

a   Reexamination of the same infants.
b   Vacuum extraction.
c   Spontaneous delivery.

8th day 85% of the haemorrhages had disappeared. Doege (1969) found 50% dissolved after 4 days, and after 3 weeks mainly macular haermorrhages were still visible. Pommer (1972) reports on 140 eyes with haemorrhages, 60% of which were dissolved after 3 days, and none of which visible after 8 days.

Submembranacious haemorrhages are of possible clinical significance with their slow resorption, tissue damage and frequent central position. Duke-Elder (1967) thought that granular haemorrhages of the internal granular layer also resorb slowly. This does not hold true according to our examinations, at least not for perinatal retinal haemorrhages.

Some original observations concerning resorption are given with the text of the plates. It is remarkable that extensive flat haemorrhages can disappear entirely within a few days. Even more surprising was the entire resorption of one particular submembranacious haemorrhage (Plate II) within 5 days! This is not the rule. Normally they persist for weeks. Tadashi and Fujimori (1941) found relics of such a haemorrhage after 45 days; Wille (1946) published 2–3 months as a resorption time; Neuweiler and Onwudiwe (1967), up to 3 months; Sezen (1970), 6 weeks. Brandstrup (1969) thinks that only those haemorrhages covering the macula for weeks can be of clinical significance.

The onset of resorption in flat haemorrhages is visible as their margins become more indistinct. Tranou-Sphalangakou (1968) also reports of resorption from the centres. Belmonte-Gonzales (1947) thinks that the centripetal resorption finally uncovers the source of bleeding. This seems doubtful, since haemorrhages can spread very excentrically from the original vessel rupture.

C. Postnatal Extension

Even with general agreement about the quick resorption of perinatal retinal haemorrhages, there is a report by Duke-Elder that flat haemorrhages can spread considerably within half an hour. This seems to be cited from the extraordinary case reported by Belmonte-Gonzales (1947), who reexamined every 5 min and saw a haemorrhage close to the disc spreading within 30 min so far that the posterior half of the fundus was occupied. Unfortunately nothing is said about the coagulation time in this child. Fundus photographs of extensive haemorrhages prove that many different sources of bleeding cause a confluent layer of blood. Therefore, it is difficult to imagine how a single source of bleeding close to the disc should cause spreading of a haemorrhage far distant along nerve fibres and not detach the internal limiting membrane.

Another unusual observation is that of Evsyukova (1969), who in her short communication reports on the spread of perinatal haemorrhages until up to the 5th day and, in cases of asphyxia, even until up to 14–18 days. The only other similar report is that by Kozuhowska (1954), who observed children 6 h after birth. In a series of 310 children, 84 had retinal haemorrhages, several of which became larger with further observation and 5 of these latter markedly. Two of these children had a pathologic coagulation time. No fundus photographs have been taken of these observations.

Certainly the haemorrhages must spread for a while until the fibrin thrombus occludes the vessel and, even after that moment, the blood cells still penetrate surrounding areas. This is supported greatly by the photographic and planimetric observations by Baum and Bulpitt (1970). They found a limited spread of two out of ten haemorrhages at the 1st day, but otherwise confirmed the generally observed quick resorption of haemorrhages. This very precise report, like that of Giles, who saw the children immediately after birth, makes it very unlikely that a true postnatal expansion of the haemorrhages occurs. Other authors, too, who reexamined the children, did not observe anything of this order (Falls and Jurow, 1946; Wille, 1946; Cavrot, 1956; Puskás and Szabó, 1962).

D. Summary

The haemorrhages occur during labour. A postnatal expansion remains doubtful. There is general agreement that the flat haemorrhages resorb quickly, whereas submembranacious haemorrhages can resorb within a few days or be visible after weeks or months.

Zusammenfassung

Die Netzhautblutungen entstehen unter der Geburt. Eine postnatale Größenzunahme wird nur in einigen, anzweifelbaren Berichten erwähnt. Übereinstimmend ist beobachtet worden, daß die Blutungen sich schnell verkleinern bzw. resorbiert werden. Nur submembranöse Kugelblutungen haben eine längere Resorptionszeit, die zwischen Tagen und Wochen schwankt.

VI. Numerical Data

A. Quantitative Evaluation

1. Literature

The fundus of newborn infants can demonstrate a wide range of haemorrhages, from a single hardly visible linear extravasation to massive confluent extravasations covering the major part of the posterior fundus. Several authors tried to quantify these haemorrhages in order to relate number of haemorrhages to the often-discussed clinical significance.

Franceschetti and Balavoine (1951) and Weiden (1970) subdivided the haemorrhages into a light and a severe group. Maumenee et al. (1941) and Pajor et al. (1964) subdivided into four groups. Most other authors use expressions like light, medium, heavy (Wille, 1946; Maertens and Götz, 1967). A small table according to this classification can be drawn up from the literature (Table 4).

Table 4. Incidence of different degrees of retinal haemorrhages

Author	Year	Retinal haemorrhages		
		Light	Medium	Severe
Ko	1924	8.7%	5.4%	10.0%
Mayer and Maria	1952	10.4%	11.4%	8.8%
Cavrot	1956	29	9	46
Ishikawa	1959	54.1%	30.1%	15.8% [a]
Panagiotou et al.	1968	230	10 [a]	53 [b]

a   Related to 100% of haemorrhages found.
b   Quantitative classification: up to 5; 5—9; many haemorrhages.

Other authors classify according to the number of haemorrhages counted, thus Takeda (1968): Up to 10 haemorrhages, 10—20, and more than 20 haemorrhages; Tranou-Sphalangakou (1968): 1—5 haemorrhages, 5—10, numerous haemorrhages, and haemorrhages within the entire posteriour half of the fundus. The subdivision of Kobayashi et al. (1964) is similar: 1—5 haemorrhages, 6—10 haemorrhages, more than 11 haemorrhages.

The results from different authors, even with attempted numerical classification, seem to be incompatible. Certainly individual judgements about severity of haemorrhage make Table 4 rather valueless.

2. Numerical Classification Applied Here

Not to overemphasize the importance of numerical classification, but for a greater degree of exactitude in this series, the number of haemorrhages and their location were noted. As quantitative subdivisions five groups were formed:

1. No retinal haemorrhage. In this group venous dilatation and sometimes indistinct papillary borders were observed but were not taken into further consideration.

2. 1–3 haemorrhages. Normally small linear haemorrhages of the nerve fibre layer, rarely isolated flame-shaped haemorrhages.

3. 4–10 haemorrhages. Normally linear and several flat haemorrhages.

4. 11–20 haemorrhages. Predominantly flat haemorrhages of the nerve fibre and granular layers, also submembranacious haemorrhages occurring in this group.

5. More than 20 haemorrhages. This is the group of the "thrombosis-like" haemorrhages, with many visible sources of bleeding in confluent development of the haemorrhages.

   In some cases more than 50 white fibrin thrombi could be counted, so that a further subdivision was not attempted. Submembranacious haemorrhages are mainly encountered in this group, though not entirely dependent on the number of haemorrhages.

   On the basis of the 200 observed "normal cases" the distribution between the different groups for 400 eyes is shown in Table 5.

Table 5. Number of haemorrhages according to numerical groups (400 eyes)

Group	Haemorrhages	Eyes
a	0	279
b	1– 3	21
c	4–10	38
d	11–20	25
e	21 and more	37

In general the distribution of haemorrhages was fairly symmetric. When it was not, the eyes of a pair fell into groups separated by one step, or rarely by two steps. The greatest discrepancy, i.e. massive haemorrhages on one side and no haemorrhages on the other, was found in four cases. These findings point to individual anatomic variants in the vessel systems draining the central retinal vein and the patency of the optic sheaths (cf. Chap. VII, Sect. E).

It has been mentioned that a classification according to the location is clinically possibly more significant, i.e. macular involvement by submembranacious haemorrhages.

3. Summary

Many different degrees of retinal involvement of perinatal haemorrhages can be distinguished. Though a classification according to macular involvement might be more important for the evaluation of different types of delivery, a quantitative classification may be of some value too. The material of this series has been classified into five groups ranging from no haemorrhages to more than 20 haemorrhages.

Zusammenfassung

Viele Grade von Netzhautbeteiligung können bei perinatalen Blutungen unterschieden werden. Um verschiedene Geburtsverläufe zu bewerten, würde eine Klassifikation je nach dem Befall der Macula am wichtigsten sein, eine quantitative Einteilung kann jedoch ebenfalls von gewissem Wert sein. Das eigene Material wurde auch nach der Anzahl der Blutungen klassifiziert und in 5 Gruppen eingeteilt: Keine Blutungen bis über 20 Blutungen.

B. Incidence

In all papers on the clinical importance of perinatal haemorrhages, the incidence of retinal haemorrhages found is a standard item. The differences in the groups examined, examination dates and techniques, cause considerable discrepancy between the results from different authors. In order to avoid conclusions from series that are too small, the voluminous literature on aetiologic factors has been studied and a survey will be presented in the following chapter. The total incidence will be discussed now, whatever its importance might be.

1. Histology

As regards the incidence in post mortem series, we have to go back to the early authors: Naumoff (1890) saw 12 pairs of eyes with haemorrhages (25.5%) in 47 mature infants who died at birth or shortly after. He found no retinal haemorrhages in 22 immature infants of the same series. Von Hippel (1898): 24 eyes, 10 with haemorrhages. Coburn (1904): 37 children, 17 with haemorrhages.

Presumably the incidences of haemorrhages will not be parallel in the group of children dying after birth and the other group of healthy children. But even the histologic series seem to be too different to be compared: Lachmann (1927) found haemorrhages in only 5 cases out of 73 stillborn infants or infants who had died after birth. It is not clear whether these infants were immature and whether serial sections were used to look for haemorrhages. The percentage in Jacobs (1928) is much higher, with 14 children, 12 of whom had retinal haemorrhages. But here it cannot be denied that retinal haemorrhages were due to the fatal intracranial haemorrhages, at least in some of his cases.

2. Clinical Observations

This involves comparing some very dissimilar statistics! Every clinical series seems to culminate in one figure, the overall incidence of retinal haemorrhages. regardless of how this was obtained and on what this was based. The largest table in the literature is from Takeda (1968), citing 47 authors. From the material compiled for this monograph a similar table of many more than 100 authors could be arranged, but this would be pointless. For instance, the extreme values of these typical tables are based on wrong quotations. On the one hand the minimum attributed to Chase et al. of 2.6% haemorrhages (as cited, e.g. by Schenker and Gombos, 1966; Brogi et al., 1962; Wierhake, 1971) is misleading. Normally one tries to compare the results of first-day examinations. In this case the figure of Chase et al. would be 8%, since they saw only 26 children on the first day and found 2 with haemorrhages. Their overall incidence of 2.6% is lower because of the late examination date. Beyond that, their figures are further discredited by the fact that they tried to examine 1241 children but could see the fundus well enough in only 839. Another minimal figure of 3% is reported by Luptakova (1972), but she was unable to judge the macular area in 27% of 503 children.

On the other hand, the maximum of 50% retinal haemorrhages from Vancea (cited by Chase et al., 1950; Yoshioka, 1954; Brogi et al., 1962; Pannarale, 1966; Duke-Elder, 1967) is also wrong. Vancea (1941) reports about 11.8% haemorrhages. The source for the wrong quotation remains unclear.

The reason for the remaining discrepancy is seen mainly in the late examination date (cf. Table 3). The first examination was done as late as the 3rd day by Murillo and Murillo (7.78% haemorrhages), up to the 4th day by Mijares (6.6%) and Critchley (13%), up to the 5th day by Vancea (11.8%), up to the 6th day by Rowland (2.75%) and Veinbaum (3.2%), up to the 7th day by Duhard and Pages (5.3%), and finally up to the 8th day with the otherwise important work of Frances Richman (12.2%). With this group of authors, a low incidence can be explained by the date of examination. With others, the reason is unclear (Bedell, 1924; Powelett and Townes, 1948; Glawanakowa et al., 1968; Martinez and Grom, 1969). With Blanc (1967) and Chosson (1967), it remains questionable whether the pupils were dilated. Critchley (1968) and Zgorzalewicz et al. (1975) did not dilate them.

Considerable discrepancies must arise from the incompatible groups examined. Thus, e.g. Gajaria et al. (1965) had only 29 primiparae among 200 cases. Giles (1960) saw 57 cases of forceps delivery among 100 children, Fritz et al. (1966), mainly children after vacuum extraction; Baum and Bulpitt (1970), more than 50% premature infants. Anaesthesia was used in more than 50% of the cases in Zisa et al. (1975).

While it might be more generous to explain the variations in incidence in terms of the dates of examination and the differences between the groups examined, the author believes the quality of examination to be the most important factor. However, the difficulties must not be overlooked. Comparing the numerical evaluation of this investigation based on indirect opthalmoscopy with fundus photographs, it was obvious that some of the finest linear extravasations (Fig. 59) simply had not been counted. Then, too, the post mortem examination of the retina reveals haemorrhages so minute that they could well have been overlooked in funduscopic examination. Similarly in all steps between the smallest, barely visible extravasations to larger ones that cannot be overlooked, the figures published in the literature would only represent minimal figures.

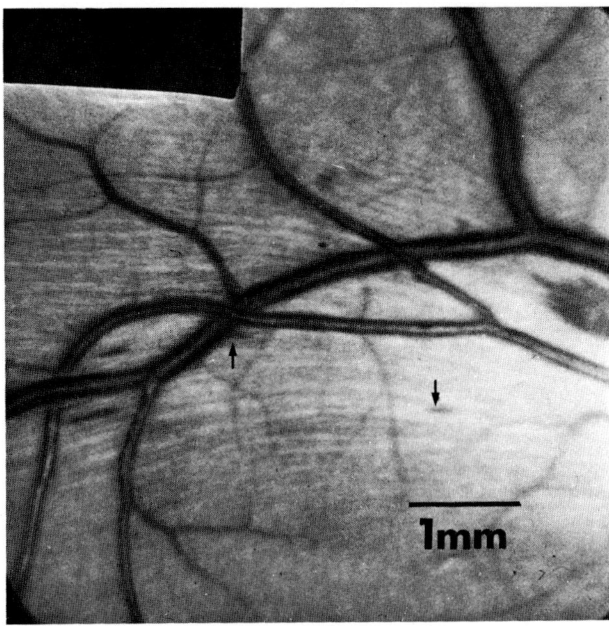

Fig. 59. Detail from Plate II. Besides flame-shaped haemorrhage at right border, photograph reveals extremely fine linear haemorrhages of nerve fibre layer of a length of 200 μm (*arrows*). One of these situated at crossing of superior temporal artery and vein. Minute haemorrhages like these are easily overlooked and are better traced on fundus photographs

Direct ophthalmoscopy is difficult because of the frequent eye movements of the newborn infants. Indirect ophthalmoscopy was recommended by Casanovas et al. (1959), Honegger (1969) and Weiden (1970). Certainly, areas beyond the centre have not been properly seen in many examinations, as is demonstrated by the remarks (Cavrot, 1956; Moulène, 1965) or the fundus drawings (de Freitas and Garcia, 1968; Murillo and Murillo, 1968) of some authors. This is not meant to indicate that the peripheral haemorrhages were of special significance, but merely to point out how little value many papers have for the estimation of the overall incidence of retinal haemorrhages. Values under 15% seem to be less reliable. Braendstrup (1969) estimates the general incidence of retinal haemorrhages at 50%, after 10 years as a consultant at a children's hospital. Wierhake's 39%, based on fundus photographs, seems to be very reliable. Taking into account different types of delivery, the author's series would also have a total incidence of 40%. In conclusion, the overall incidence of retinal haemorrhage, found with careful examination within the first 24 h of a comparatively "normal" group of infants, would be at least 1/3.

Racial differences seem to be neglibigle. Sykes (1931) and Kauffman (1941) found black and white babies with the same incidence of haemorrhages. The Japanese publications do not indicate that the incidence there is different from Caucasian groups.

3. Summary

About 1/3 or more of all newborn infants present perinatal retinal haemorrhages. Although the incidence of perinatal haemorrhage is not very important, many authors have tried to compile a series of overall figures to compare their material with the material of others. Differences in examination dates, in group composition according to aetiologic factors and in examination quality, are the bases for the contradiction in total figures, which makes the different publications incompatible.

Zusammenfassung

Ungefähr 1/3 aller Neugeborenen hat perinatale Netzhautblutungen. Obwohl die Blutungshäufigkeit als solche nicht sehr wichtig ist, haben viele Autoren versucht, ihre Ergebnisse mit den Serien anderer Autoren zu vergleichen. Verschiedene Untersuchungsdaten, Gruppenzusammensetzungen nach ätiologischen Faktoren und zweifellos auch Unterschiede in der Untersuchungsqualität verursachen die starken Widersprüche der Gesamtzahlen, so daß die verschiedenen Publikationen nicht vergleichbar sind.

VII. Aetiology

Königstein's first description of this type of haemorrhage also comprised the first speculation on its origin. A great number of subsequent authors tried to solve the problem from many different points of view. Since there is not one invididual factor which explains perinatal retinal haemorrhage, and since many series studied were too small for a proper evaluation, the results obtained are in considerable disagreement. To evaluate the different factors discussed in connection with perinatal haemorrhage an extensive review of the literature is given and comparisons are made with the observations in our series. Thus, from the multitude of factors presumed to cause these haemorrhages it may be possible to select a few more important ones.

A. Types of Delivery

Without any doubt, different types of delivery have a definite influence on incidence and intensity of retinal haemorrhage. This was observed by Paul (1900), who found a doubled incidence of haemorrhage in complicated delivery.

1. Spontaneous Delivery from Occipital Presentation

a) General Data

The normal course of delivery, which occurs in 95% of all cases (Martius, 1971) is spontaneous delivery from occipital presentation. Thus, to analyse the influence of other types of labour and other factors, this most frequent type of delivery must be considered first.

Very often, in the literature, only the overall incidence of haemorrhage is noted, including factors that elevate it – like vacuum extraction – or decrease it – like caesarian section. More useful in comparing the incidence reported by different authors would be a table dealing with only spontaneous delivery. References have been compiled in Table 6. Differences remain in examination time and certainly, as mentioned before, in examination quality.

Examining the children within 1 h after birth, Giles (1960) found haemorrhage in 34% of the cases after spontaneous delivery. The figure of 40.6% reported by Wierhake is based on fundus photographs of 1st and 2nd days. In the author's series, the incidence is 39%. Disregarding other factors (e.g. duration of second stage of labour, asphyxia), the incidence of haemorrhage after spontaneous delivery from occipital presentation seems to be at least 1/3.

Table 6. Incidence of retinal haemorrhages after spontaneous delivery from occiptal presentation

Author	Year	Date of examination [a]	Cases	Haemorrhages	Percent
Sykes	1931	1	61	282	21
Edgerton	1934	2	118	402	29.6
Belmonte	1947	2	23	86	26
Chase et al.	1950	3	13	627	2.1
Grassi and Musini	1950	1	37	264	14
Millán and Beltrán	1950	2	10	71	14
Franceschetti and Balavoine	1951	2	564		14.9
Štefek	1951	2			16
Kozuhowska	1954	1	75	284	26.4
Nevinny-Stickel	1954		47	124	38
Tóspelas and Charamis	1955	1	31	135	22.96
Cavrot	1956	2	50	316	15.8
Konstantopais	1956	1	43	159	27
Lomičková and Otradovec	1956	2	131	462	28.3
Singer et al.	1956	2			18.75
Lemmingson and Stark	1957	2	74	264	28
Koyama	1959		105	409	25.7
Fulst	1960	3	57	265	21.5
Giles	1960	1	16	47	34
Motohashi and Kobayashi	1960	1	39	179	21.2
Puskás and Sazbó	1961	1	60	228	26.3
Yohitda et al.	1961	1	105	409	25.7
Kawakami et al.	1963	1	71	380	18.68
Sanchez-Ibanez et al.	1963	1	109	324	33.6
Kobayashi et al.	1964	3	23	102	22.6
Treit et al.	1964	2	45	225	17
Jain and Gupta	1965	3	36	134	26.9
Krauer-Meyer	1965	3	106		20.5
Moulene	1965	2	30	95	31.57
Pannarale	1966	2	99	378	26
Maertens and Götz	1967	1	27	87	31
Neuweiler and Onwudiwe	1967	1	903		34.8
Takala and Sopanen	1967	1	61	211	28.9
Bachmann et al.	1968	3	103	438	23.5
Buchhalter and Schnecke	1968	1	200		31
Panagiotou et al.	1968	2	165	745	22
Takeda	1968	1	80	345	23.1
Tranou-Sphalangakou	1968	3	56	189	29.5
Hickl et al.	1969	1	19	50	38
Lukaszewicz and Zaporowski	1969	1	30	94	32
Richter	1969	?	918		18
Vincenti and Gavinelli	1969	1	13	101	12.87
Baum and Bulpitt	1970	3	24	109	22
Sezen	1970	3	147	1042	14.2
Planten and v.d. Schaaf	1971	1	34	154	22
Wierhake	1971	2	106	261	40.6
von Barsewisch	1972	1	78	200	39
Pommer	1972	1	91	668	14
Zisa et al.	1975	1	87	836	10.4

a Date of examination: 1, seen within 24 h
              2, within the first 2 days
              3, first seen later than the 2nd day.

b) Number and Location

From our material even the number of haemorrhages can be precisely deduced. Out of 200 cases. 78 had haemorrhaging and, arranged according to the more affected eye, the incidence in the different groups is shown in Table 7.

Table 7. Number of haemorrhages in 200 cases

Group	Haemorrhages	Cases
a	0	122
b	1– 3	12
c	4–10	23
d	11–20	19
e	more than 20	24

In other words, 12% of the cases had extensive haemorrhages at least in one eye. These were also the cases with macular involvement. Here the fovea was covered in 8 children (9 eyes) and, in another 12 children (19 eyes), the haemorrhage extended to the macular area.

c) Left or Right Occipital Presentation

Stumpf and Sicherer (1909) found a marked asymmetric distribution according to left or right occipital presentation in 40 cases with haemorrhage. A few other authors reported on this correlation (Duesberg and Tiburtius, 1958; Fulst, 1960; Nevinny-Stickel, 1954). More detailed information was given by only nine authors (Table 8). The result seems to be a rather random distribution of haemorrhage and no correlation of one side or the other with left or right occipital presentation. Nor, in the author's material of 311 children (including the series with fibrinolysis inhibitor) and 131 haemorrhages, is any correlation with either presentation to be seen. Kauffman (1941), too, found no preference for one side in his material of 3381 children.

2. Forceps delivery

Two groups have to be distinguished: Injuries by forceps delivery and retinal haemorrhages after normal forceps delivery. "Haemorrhages due to forceps delivery" is a misleading expression. It seems far more likely that the conditions that led to a termination of the birth by forceps are the causes for retinal haemorrhage.

a) Forceps Injuries

At the beginning of this century, traumatic sequelae of forceps deliveries played a major role. Ophthalmic lesions, sometimes with retinal haemorrhages, were mentioned by de Wecker (1926). Histologic descriptions of such traumatic retinal haemorrhages lend the communications of Wintersteiner (1899), Peters (1907) and Rupprecht (1908) a certain degree of interest.

Table 8. Lateral distribution of retinal haemorrhages in relation to left or right occipital presentation

Author	Year	Examination date	Number of cases	With retinal haemorrhages	Left or right occipital presentation	Cases	With retinal haemorrhages	Predominantly right	Equal in both eyes	Predominantly left	Remarks
Stumpf and v. Sicherer	1909	1	200	42	l		28	21	5	2	
					r		12	2	3	7	
Jacobs	1924	2	190	23	l		6	2	4	0	
					r		11	5	3	3	
Juler	1926	3	158	14	l	29	7	3	2	2	
					r	20	3	1	2	0	
Edgerton	1934	2	458	191	l	313	93	31	44	18	
					r	89	25	8	7	10	
Štefek	1951	2			l			28%	36%	36%	
					r			26%	39%	35%	
Terado	1953	1	88	28	l	48		14		18	a
					r	35		11		11	
Koyama	1959	1	510	133	l	265	67	24	30	13	
					r	245	53	13	36	17	
Gajaria et al.	1965	1	200	43	l		20	14		6	
					r		4	2		2	
Neuweiler and Onwudiwe	1967	1	1074	357	l	348	147	73		74	
					r	310	129	65		64	
Takeda	1968	1	552	141	l		56	18	22	16	
					r		51	11	25	15	
von Barsewisch	1972	1	311	131	l	135	98	32	34	32	
					r	78	33	12	9	12	

a   Bilateral haemorrhages seem to have been counted twice.

b) Retinal Haemorrhages After Forceps Delivery

Obstetric techniques have changed considerably, so that difficult forceps delivery has been replaced by caesarian section, and vacuum extraction competes with "normal" forceps delivery.

For the discussion of different obstetric techniques in the following sections, the actual point of view of obstetricians must be taken into consideration. Martius (1965) reported on perinatal mortality in 243 obstetric interventions. If intervention for the sake of the mother was necessary, the mortality was 0. If intervention for the sake of the child was necessary, the overall mortality was 3.7% (caesarian section, 4.1%, forceps delivery, 3.3% and vacuum extraction, 2.1%). Perinatal asphyxia is more dangerous to the foetus than mechanical birth trauma. Obstetric vaginal operations in themselves are not hazardous to the foetus if no hypoxic damage has yet occurred. The rest of the chapter has to be considered with these points in mind.

The comparison between spontaneous delivery and forceps delivery has been discussed in the literature since the 1930s. The result is given in Table 9. In this table, the incidence is very low only with Murillo and Murillo, possibly because of the late examination date. For the others, the absolute figures cannot be compared and, as mentioned before, an average cannot be calculated. Only comparing the figures of each author, obtained under the same conditions, can a certain tendency be found. A few authors (Mayer and Maria, 1952; Sanchez-Ibanez et al., 1963; Casanovas et al., 1959) found less haemorrhaging after forceps delivery than after spontaneous delivery from occipital presentation. For the rest, the incidence of haemorrhage is higher after forceps delivery, sometimes twice as high compared with normal birth. On average the incidence is greater by a factor of 1.5. In the author's series, only four children were seen after forceps delivery, two with haemorrhages — a figure too small to be significant.

Unfortunately, there are few reports on the intensity of retinal haemorrhage after forceps delivery. Edgerton found that all 17 children after high forceps delivery had bilateral haemorrhage as opposed to those delivered by low forceps, with 50% bilateral haemorrhage. Puskás and Szabó found severe haemorrhages in 3 out of 60 children after normal birth and 3 out of 5 after forceps delivery. Practically the same tendency is reported by Koyama: 405 spontaneous deliveries with three macular haemorrhages; 71 forceps deliveries with six macular haemorrhages.

The reason for the use of forceps is hardly ever given in detail. Millán and Beltrán (1950) report that about half their forceps deliveries were occasioned by intrauterine asphyxia. Of the 18 haemorrhages they found, 15 were from this group, i.e. 5/6 of the infants with haemorrhage were delivered by forceps because of intrauterine asphyxia. This same cause would be involved in most of the other series, as Naumoff (1890) wrote: "Operations are usually performed in cases where conditions are present that promote the occurrence of alterations on foetal eyes".

3. Vacuum Extraction

Evelbauer reported a first series of 50 cases in 1956. In 1963 he was able to report on 580 cases from 8 years' experience. During this time use of forceps was reduced to 0.1%, whereas the vacuum extractor was used in 9.6% of 6031 births. The incidence of caesarian section remained practically unaltered at 10.5%.

Table 9. Incidence of retinal haemorrhages after forceps delivery.

Author	Year	Examination date	Spontaneous delivery, occipital presentation			Forceps delivery			Remarks
			Ret. Haem.	Cases	%	Ret. Haem.	Cases	%	
Ko	1924	?	36	114	32	2	4	50	
Sykes	1931	1	61	282	21	10	24	41	
Edgerton	1934	2	118	402	30	17	17	100	a
						58	95	61	b
Rico	1939	3	19	100	19	2	8	75	c
Kauffman	1941	3	398	2331	17	31	74	42	a
						11	36	31	b
McKeown	1941	3			42	86	148	58	
Belmonte Gonzales	1947	2	23	86	26	8	14	57	
Jarny	1947	2	11	50	22	5	25	20	
Chase et al.	1950	3	13	627	2	9	178	5	
Grassi and Musini	1950	1	37	264	14	4	24	16	
Millán and Beltrán	1950	2	10	71	14	18	55	33	
Franceschetti and Balavoine	1951	2		564	15		13	23	a
Štefek	1951	2			16		7	42	b
Mayer and Maria	1952	1		?	36			27	
Tsópelas and Charamis	1955	1	31	135	23	4	15	27	
Lomičková and Otradovec	1956	2	131	462	28	4	9	45	
Singer et al.	1956				19			24	
Lemmingson and Stark	1957	2	74	264	28	6	16	38	
Cordero and Najul	1958	?	46	389	12	16	16	100	d
Casanovas et al.	1959	1			35		35	22	
Koyama	1959		105	409	26	27	71	38	
Mao	1959	2			15			29	
Giles	1960	1	16	47	34	24	53	45	
Motohashi and Kobayashi	1960	1	39	179	21	3	7	43	
Puskás and Szabó	1961	1	60	228	26	5	13	38	
Yohitda et al.	1961	1	105	409	26	27	71	38	

Sanchez-Ibanez et al.	1963	1	109	324	34	4	13	31	
Treit et al.	1964	2	42	225	17	2	8	75	
Jain and Gupta	1965	3	36	134	27	3	11	28	
Konstantopais	1965	1	43	159	27	2	8	25	
Krauer-Meyer	1965	3	17	101	17	14	50	28	
Aliquò-Mazzei	1966	2?	11	50	22	2	5	40	
Pannarale	1966	2	99	378	26	40	80	50	
Schenker and Gombos	1966	1			19		16	31	
Neuweiler and Onwudiwe	1967	1		903	35		42	43	
Gombos and Schenker	1967	1	42	244	18	9	25	36	e
Bachmann et al.	1968	3	103	438	24	6	9	67	
Murillo and Murillo	1968	3		0		6	231	3	
Panagiotou et al.	1968	2	165	745	22	22	59	37	
Martinez and Grom	1969	1		0		22	102	22	f
Richter	1969	?		918	18		32	10	
Vincenti and Gavinelli	1969	1	13	101	13	4	11	36	
Baum and Bulpitt	1970	3	24	109	22	8	12	67	g
Orduña and De Arizcun	1970	2	13	71	18	31	102	30	
Sezen	1970	3	142	1042	14	3	9	33	
Planten and v.d. Schaaf	1971	1	34	154	22	5	23	22	
Wierhake	1971	2	106	261	41	3	6	50	
Pommer	1972	1	91	668	14	4	12	33	
Ciechanowska et al.	1974	1?		132	17		4	100	
Ehlers et al.	1974	1	57	207	28	38	99	38	
Krause et al.	1974	2	101	500	20	3	10	30	
Zisa et al	1975	1	87	836		10	37		
Bergen and Margolis	1976	1	13	38	34	20	41	40	

a High forceps.
b Low forceps.
c Total series.
d No primiparae.
e 22 because of foetal asphyxia.
f 102 with occipital presentation, 22 haemorrhages including 6 vitreous haemorrhages.
g Mainly premature infants.

Table 10. Incidence of retinal haemorrhages after vacuum extraction

Author	Year	Examination date	Spontaneous delivery from occipital presentation			Vacuum extraction		
			Ret. haem.	Cases	%	Ret. haem.	Cases	%
Voegeli	1958		5	89		4	89	
Fulst	1960	3	57	265	22	13	65	20
high vacuum extr.						7	1	
low vacuum extr.						58	12	
de Azevedo et al.	1963	1	5	44	11	6	25	24
Kawakami et al.	1963	1	71	380	11	20	62	32
Sanchez-Ibanez	1963	1	109	324	34	32	54	59
Treit et al.	1964	2	42	255	17	10	55	18
Krauer-Meyer	1965	3	17	101	17	35	53	66
Moulène	1965	2	30	95	32	29	50	58
Aliquò-Mazzei	1966	2?	11	50	22	20	50	40
Krebs and Jäger	1966	3		?	20		22	41
Schenker and Gombos	1966	1		?			25	52
Gombos and Schenker	1967	1	42	244	18	31	59	52
Maertens and Götz	1967	1	27	87	31	17	23	74
Neuweiler and Onwudiwe	1967	1		903	35		29	72
Takala and Sopanen	1967	1	61	211	29	11	67	52
Bachmann et al.	1968	3	103	438	24	55	110	50
Bruniquel and Dollard	1968	2	3	46	5	6	56	11
Buchhalter and Schnecke	1968	1		200	31		98	49
Murillo and Murillo	1968	3		0		1	10	10
Stefanini et al.	1968	1	10	52	19	22	42	48
Takeda	1968	1	80	345	23	23	63	37
Tranou-Sphalangakou	1968	3	56	189	30	46	141	33
Hickl et al.	1969	1	19	50	38	45	77	58
Nordentoft and Dalsgård	1969	1		?			?	64
Richter	1969	?		918	18		11	46
Santamarina	1969	1		?		6	26	23

Vincenti and Gavinelli	1969	1	13	103	13	3	11	18
Orduña and De Arizcun	1970	2		?		14	25	56
Sezen	1970	3	147	1042	14	25	62	40
Loriaux and Toussaint	1971	1	17	127	13	48	18	38
Planten and Schaaf	1971	1	34	154	22	8	20	40
Schlaeder et al.	1971	3	29	198	15	27	65	42
Wierhake	1971	2	106	261	41	6	11	55
v. Barsewisch	1972	1	78	200	39	19	26	73
Hoo	1973	1	18	100	18	45	100	45
Ciechanowska et al.	1974	1?		132	17		52	48
Ehlers et al.	1974	1	57	207	28	60	94	64
Krause et al.	1974	2	101	500	20	12	25	48
Zgorzalewicz	1975	1	15	100	15	42	110	38

The indications for vacuum extraction were classified in four different groups:

A) Maternal (e.g. organic disease, fever, etc.)
B) Foetal (e.g. asphyxia, prolapse of the umbilical cord, etc.)
C) Special and prophylactic (e.g. protracted course of labour, preceding caesarian section, twins, special presentations, etc.)
D) Specific vacuum (cases too late for caesarian section and too early for forceps delivery).

Of his cases where vacuum extraction was used, 28.5% were due to protacted course of labour and 26.1% to intrauterine asphyxia. This again hints at the importance of predisposing factors causing haemorrhages in cases where vacuum extraction is resorted to.

The statistics relative to Evelbauer's series were published by Fulst (1960), based on a rather late examination date. The incidence of haemorrhage was very low in that series. The first series published by Voegeli (1958) also reports an incidence that is incomprehensible, far below all other authors'. More data from the literature are compiled in Table 10.

Absolute figures are not obtainable even from this extensive table. As with forceps delivery, it is possible to estimate only the relation between rates of heamorrhage in spontaneous delivery and vacuum extraction. The incidence of haemorrhage increases with vacuum extraction by a factor of 1.5 to 2 if one compares the figures of each author.

Ehlers et al. (1974) made a random selection to compare retinal haemorrhages after forceps (38%) with those after vacuum extraction (64%). With 13 infants vacuum extraction had been carried out after an attempt with forceps. Of these, 9 had haemorrhages. The duration of traction was found to be influential by Schenker and Gombos(1966) and Schlaeder et al. (1971), the intensity of traction by Krauer (1965), the number of times traction was applied, by Zgorzalewicz (1975). Bruniquel and Dollard (1968) recommend measuring the force of traction in order to avoid values exceeding 7 kg.

Not only the incidence but also the intensity of retinal haemorrhages were found increased after vacuum extraction (Krauer-Meier, 1965a; Hickl et al., 1969; Nordentoft and Dalsgård, 1969; Weiden, 1970; Schlaeder et al., 1971; Zgorzalewicz, 1975).

Our series includes 26 vacuum extractions (not part of the series of fibrinolysis inhibitors). Among these, there were 19 cases with haemorrhages, 10 of which had massive bilateral extravasations (i.e. more than 20). Macular involvement was present in nine eyes of these seven children, and submembranacious haemorrhages were present in seven eyes of six children. Our material was too small to be classified according to the indication for vacuum extraction. Possibly the incidence was so high because vacuum extraction was mainly performed due to foetal indication. A second stage of labour lasting more than 30 min was present in half the cases with vacuum extraction, whereas in the normal series it was only present in 1/10. The mean time of birth in the series of Bachmann et al. (1968) was 12.6 h, i.e. about twice as long as in spontaneous deliveries. Stefanini et al. (1968) compare the cases of vacuum extraction with hypoxia (20 infants, 14 with haemorrhages = 70%) to those without hypoxia (26 infants, 8 with haemorrhages = 31%).

Although indications differ in different hospitals, in most cases vacuum extraction should not be looked upon as causing retinal haemorrhages (Krebs and Jaeger, 1966). The connection is rather to be found in the factors that indicated vacuum-extraction (Schlaeder et al., 1971).

4. Caesarian Section

After some single cases had been published, Stocker (1927) reported on 22 cases of infants seen within the first day after caesarian section. None of these had retinal haemorrhages. The correlation has been confirmed by a large group of observers, and the references have been gathered in Table 11. Again, no average can be calculated from the series, many of which are very small. On the whole, the incidence of retinal haemorrhage is about 5%. Differences are due mainly to different obstetric techniques. Thus, for example. all five children in the series of Moulène had haemorrhages after caesarian section, but the section was performed only after an attempted spontaneous delivery. There are more reports about the operation having been executed only in cases of intrauterine asphyxia or after attempted spontaneous delivery (Belmonte-Gonzales, 1947; Jirman, 1947; Millán and Beltrán, 1950; Lomičková and Otradovec, 1956; Pannarale, 1966; Neuweiler and Onwudiwe, 1967). Other authors state that if retinal haemorrhages occurred they were not severe (Edgerton, 1934; Franceschetti and Balavoine, 1951; Puskás and Szabó, 1961).

Our series comprises eight children seen after caesarian section. Three of them had retinal haemorrhages:

1. One single linear haemorrhage (indication for operation: previous caesarian section)
2. One single, small, flame-shaped haemorrhage in the periphery (indication: contracted pelvis)
3. Heavy bilateral haemorrhages (foetal indication: asphyxia)

Of course this group is too small for a statistical evaluation. The observations are in accordance with the literature, indicating that haemorrhages are either not severe or that they occur when damage to the foetus is imminent or already present.

5. Breech Presentation

With delivery from breech presentation, the head is compressed after the other parts of the body are no longer exposed to pressure. This situation causes different haemodynamic conditions and, therefore, it is of interest that the incidence of retinal haemorrhage is low. Naturally, this relatively rare type of delivery is sparsely represented in the literature (Table 12).

A higher incidence of haemorrhages was found only by McKeown and Jain and Gupta, based on small series. Comparing the figures from series larger than 20 cases (Kauffman, 1941; Stefek, 1951; Koyama, 1959; Buchhalter and Schnecke, 1968; Pommer, 1972; Ciechanowska et al., 1974), it is correct to estimate the incidence of retinal

Table 11. Indicence of retinal haemorrhages after caesarian section

Author	Year	Examination date	Spontaneous delivery from occipital presentation			Caesarian section		Remarks
			Ret. haem.	Cases	%	Ret. haem.	Cases	
Juler	1926	3		?	15.5	0	4	a
Rowland	1927	3	11	363	3	0	5	a
Stocker	1927	1		0		0	22	
Edgerton	1934	2	118	402	29.6	3	34	
Juler	1937	?		?		0	19	b
Richman	1937	3		?	12.2	0	12	a
Rico	1939	3	19	100	19	0	2	a
Kauffman	1941	3	398	2331	27	4	88	
McKeown	1941	3	197	484	40.7	0	10	
Belmonte-Gonzales	1947	2	86	23	26	2	16	c
Jarny	1947	2	11	50	22	1	8	
Jirmán	1947	1		?	39.83	3	13	a, d
Chase et al.	1950	3	13	627	2.1	0	34	
Grassi and Musini	1950	1	37	246	14	0	8	
Millán and Beltrán	1950	2	10	71	14	2	20	e
Franceschetti and Balavoine	1951	2		564	14.9	1	33	
Štefek	1951	2			16.09	0	23	
Mayer and Maria	1952	1			35.6	1	10	f
Mezey	1952	?				0	10	
Nevinny-Stickel	1954		47	124	38	0	20	
Tsópelas and Charamis	1955	1	31	135	22.96	1	9	
Lomíčková and Otradovec	1956	2	131	462	28.3	1	17	
Lemmingson and Stark	1957	2	74	264	28	0	6	
Cordero and Najul	1958	?	46	389	12	3	18	g
Casanovas et al.	1959	1			34.6	5	22	a
Koyama	1959	1	105	409	25.7	0	9	
Mao	1959	2		?		1	10	
Fulst	1960	3	57	265	21.5	0	50	

Motohashi and Kobayashi	1960	1	39	179	21.2	0	7	
Puskás and Szabó	1961	1	60	228	26;3	7	78	
Kawakami	1963	1	71	380	18.68	0	17	
Sanchez-Ibanez et al.	1963	1	1C9	327	33.6	1	25	
Treit et al.	1964	2	42	255	17	2	20	
de Freitas	1965	3	2	38	5	0	9	
Jain and Gupta	1965	1	36	134	26.9	0	10	
Konstantopais	1965	1	42	159	27	0	10	
Moulène	1965	2	30	95	31.57	5	5	h
Aliquò-Mazzei	1966	2?	11	50	22	0	5	
Krebs and Jäger	1966	3			20	17%		
Pannarale	1966	2	99	378	26	4	92	i
Schenker and Gombos	1966	1	?			0	20	
Gombos and Schenker	1967	1	42	244	18	0	38	
Neuweiler and Onwudiwe	1967	1		903	34.8	3	100	j
Takala and Sopanen	1967	1	61	211	28.9	2	23	
Bachman et al. (cf. Weiden)	1968	3	103	438	23.5	0	19	
Buchhalter and Schnecke	1968	1		200	31	1	76	
de Freitas and Garcia	1968	1		?		0	17	
Jochmus	1968	3	42	394	10.5	1	25	k
Murillo and Murillo	1968	3		0		6	231	
Pangatiotou et al.	1968	2	165	745	22	9	154	
Stafanini et al	1968	1	10	52	19	0	5	
Takeda	1968	1	80	345	23.1	0	31	
Tranou-Sphalangakou	1968	3	56	189	29.5	3	40	
Lukaszewicz and Zaporowski	1969	1	30	94	32	0	2	
Richter	1969	?		918	18	1	20	
Santamarina	1969	1				0	4	
Vincenti and Gavinelli	1969	1	13	101	12.87	1	12	l
Baum and Bulpitt	1970	3	24	109	22	3	23	
Orduña and De Arizcun	1970	2				3	34	
Sezen	1970	3	147	1042	14.2	1	125	
Loriaux and Toussaint	1971	1	17	127	13	0	8	
Neme et al.	1971	1	43	116	37	0	15	
Planten and v.d. Schaaf	1971	1	34	154	22	2	12	

Table 11 (continued)

Author	Year	Examination date	Spontaneous delivery from occipital presentation			Caesarian section		Remarks
			Ret. haem.	Cases	%	Ret. haem.	Cases	
Schlaeder et al.	1971	3	29	198	15	0	14	
Szirmák et al.	1971	1	16	123	13	0	19	m
		2	14	118	12	1	17	n
Wierhake	1971	2	106	261	40.6	1	13	
Pommer	1972	1	91	668	14	0	5	
Taleb Bendiab	1972	2	26	78	33	5	25	h
Ciechanowska et al.	1974	1?		132	17	1	14	
Krause et al.	1974	2	101	500	20	0	17	o
Zisa	1975	1	87	836	10	2	97	
Bergen and Margolis	1976	1	13	38	34	2	11	

a Comparative figure from the total series.
b C.s. prior to onset of labour.
c C.s. after attempted spontaneous delivery of 18 and 23 h respectively.
d C.S. indicated by foetal asphyxia.
e 1 c.s. after attempted forceps, the other infant asphyctic.
f C.s. because of hypertension in the mother.
g Very few primiparae.
h All c.s. after attempted labour.
i Foetal asphyxia.
j Ret. haem. in cases with cranial compression.
k Ret. haem. with a preeclamptic case; only immature infants.
l Mother with purpura thrombocytopenica.
m Mature infants.
n Immature infants.
o 8 because of hypoxia sub partu.

haemorrhage after breech delivery at about 1/3 that of normal births with occipital presentation. Besides that, haemorrhages tend to be less extensive (Mayer and Maria, 1952; Koyama, 1959). In the author's series, only five children were seen after breech presentation, and one of them had less than 10 unilateral haemorrhages. Here, additional obstetric complications were present (manoeuvre of Veit-Smellie).

6. Other Types

For the sake of completeness, rather than because of their specific importance, further obstetric problems are mentioned in this chapter. A few authors report on podalic version (Kauffman, 1941; Belmonte-Gonzales, 1947; Kozuhowska, 1954). Extractions are mentioned by Sykes (1931), Tsópelas and Charamis (1955), Lemmingson and Stark (1957), Puskás and Szabó (1961). Expression by the manoeuvre of Kristeller was related to a slightly higher incidence of retinal haemorrhages by Štefek (1951) and Richter (1969), and a pronounced elevation in the incidence was found by Singer et al. (1956), Takeda (1968) and Neme (1972). Twins are mentioned several times, but no general conclusion can be drawn (Belmonte-Gonzales, 1947; Millán and Beltrán, 1950; Musini, 1950; Drozdowa, 1951; Dolcet-Buxeres and Ferrer-Pi, 1954; Casanovas et al., 1959; Yamanouchi, 1959; Pannarale, 1966; Santamarina, 1969; Baum and Bulpitt, 1970).

Umbilical complications are mentioned by several authors, but the definitions seem to be different. McKeown (1941) reports 498 normal cases (42.1% haemorrhages) and 24 cases with cord around the neck (91.6% haemorrhages). The comparable figures drawn from the work of Takeda (1968) are: 338 normal cases (28.4% haemorrhages) and 132 cases with cord around the neck (23.5% haemorrhages). This suggests that definitions differ. Unexpectedly, a lower incidence of haemorrhage after delivery with cord around the neck was found by Stumpf and von Sicherer (1909), de Freitas and Garcia (1968) and Wierhake (1971). Practically no difference was found by Štefek (1951) and Koyama (1959). A higher incidence was published by Rico (1939), Puskás and Szabó (1962), Kawakami et al. (1963), Jain and Gupta (1965), Moulène (1965), Sopanen (1966) and Santamarina (1969).

The prolapse of the umbilical cord seems to be more clearly defined and of greater importance; it certainly can cause asphyxia. The two cases reported by McKeown (1941) and another one with a true umbilical knot, the case of Konstantopais (1956), the case of Cordero and Najul (1958), and two of the three cases of Pannarale (1966) had retinal haemorrhages.

Pommer (1972) found a reduced incidence of retinal haemorrhage after episiotomia, especially in primiparous mothers (13% vs. 26%), Loriaux and Toussaint (1971) found no connection. Jain and Gupta (1965) report a higher incidence (60% compared to 27% in spontaneous deliveries).

Table 12. Incidence of retinal haemorrhages after delivery from breech presentation

Author	Year	Examination date	Occipital presentation			Breech presentation			Remarks
			Ret. haem.	Cases	%	Ret. haem.	Cases	%	
Ko	1924	?	36	114	32	0	2		
Rico	1939	3	19	100	19	1	5		
Kauffman	1941	3	398	2331	17	7	110	6	
McKeown	1941	3			42	8	14	57	
Jarny	1947	2	11	50	22	0	3		
Millán and Beltrán	1950	2	10	71	14	0	6		
Franceschetti and Balavoine	1951	2		564	15		16	6	
Štefek	1951	2			16	0	68		
Mayer and Maria	1952	1			36	3	13	25	
Lomíčková and Otradovec	1956	2	131	462	28	1	12	8	
Singer et al.	1956	2			19			8	
Lemmingson and Stark	1957	2	74	264	28	2	10	20	
Casanovas et al.	1959	1			(34.6)	?	10	"26.6"	a
Koyama	1959	1	105	409	26	1	21	5	b
Motohashi and Kobayashi	1960	1	39	179	21	1	7	14	
Treit et al.	1964	2	42	255	17	2	8		
Jain and Gupta	1965	3	36	134	27	2	6	33	
Konstantopais	1965	1	43	159	27	1	8	9	
Aliquò-Mazzei	1966	2?	11	50	22	0	12		
Chosson et al.	1967	1	18	350	6	1	14	7	
Gombos and Schenker	1967	1	42	244	18	2	20	10	c
Takala and Sopanen	1967	1	61	211	29	2	13	15	
Bachmann et al.	1968	3	103	438	24	3	17	18	
Buchhalter and Schnecke	1968	1		200	31		42	5	
Panagiotou et al.	1968	2	165	745	22	2	38	5	
Lukaszewicz and Zaporowski	1969	1	30	94	32	0	5		
Martinez and Grom	1969		22	102	22	0	20		d
Santamarina	1969	1			(20.4)	0	7		a
Vincenti and Gavinelli	1969	1	13	101	13	0	8		

Baum and Bulpitt	1970	3	24	109	22	1	8	13	e
Orduña and De Arizcun	1970	2		?		0	15		
Loriaux and Toussaint	1971	1	17	127	13	0	9		
Pommer	1971	1	91	668	14	1	21	5	
Schlaeder et al.	1971	3	29	198	15	0	5		
Szirmák et al.	1971	1	16	123	13	0	5		f
		2	14	118	12	0	13		g
Taleb Bendiab	1972	2	26	78	33	3	12	25	
Ciechanowska	1974	1?		132	17	1	30	3	
Zisa	1975	1	87	836	10	0	9		

a　Comparative figures from the total series.
b　Light haemorrhages only.
c　One with Apgar score 2.
d　Forceps deliveries.
e　Mainly immature infants.
f　Mature infants.
g　Immature infants.

7. Duration of Labour

a) Total Duration

Naumoff (1890) had already related a longer duration of labour to a higher incidence of retinal haemorrhage. The mean value was published by some authors. The data are collected in Table 13.

Table 13. Mean time of labour and incidence of retinal haemorrhages

Author	Year	Duration of labour		First stage	Second stage
Schleich	1890	Haem. $\emptyset$:	12 h		
		Haem. +:	slightly more than 12 h		
Stumpf and von Sicherer	1909	Haem. $\emptyset$:	15 h 18 min	14 h 12 min	66 min
		Haem. +:	16 h 15 min	15 h 18 min	47 min
Falls and Jurow	1946	Haem. $\emptyset$:	9 h		
		Haem. +:	9.8 h		
Mayer and Maria	1952	Haem. $\emptyset$:	9 h 20 min		
		Haem. 1+:	10 h		
		Haem. 2+:	10 h 50 min		
		Haem. 3+:	12 h 30 min		
Lemmingson and Stark	1957	Haem. $\emptyset$:	11.9 h		
		Haem. +:	8.6 h		
Baum and Bulpitt	1970	Haem. $\emptyset$:		8.5 h	22 min
		Haem. +:		9.9 h	13.6 min
Hoo	1973	Haem. $\emptyset$:	5 h 4 min		
		Haem. +:	7 h 30 min [a]		
		Haem. $\emptyset$:	10 h 45 min [b]		
		Haem. +:	12 h 30 min		

a Spontaneous delivery.
b Vacuum extraction.

More severe haemorrhages after long duration of labour have been observed by Mayer and Maria (1952). A higher incidence can be derived from the following authors: Mezey (1952, duration over 10 h), Krebs and Jaeger (1966, duration over 24 h), Sopanen (1966) and Belmonte (1970). Moulène (1965) divided into two groups, one under 4 h and one over 4 h and found about twice as many haemorrhages in the second group. No correlation was found by Eades (1929), Richman (1937a), Tadashi and Fujimori (1941) and Weiden (1970). In several sources the total duration of labour is broken down into more detail. These data are compared in Table 14.

Table 14. Duration of labour and incidence of retinal haemorrhages (cases with haemorrhages/total series = percent)

<table>
<tr><td rowspan="2">Author</td><td rowspan="2">Year</td><td rowspan="2">a</td><td colspan="11">Hours</td></tr>
<tr><td>1 2 3</td><td>4 5</td><td>6</td><td>7 8 9</td><td>10</td><td>11 12</td><td>13 14 15</td><td>< 18</td><td>< 24</td><td>< 30</td><td>> 30</td></tr>
<tr><td>McKeown</td><td>1941</td><td></td><td colspan="3">28%</td><td colspan="4">37%</td><td>38%</td><td>51%</td><td>90%</td><td>100%</td></tr>
<tr><td>Dolcet and Ferrer</td><td>1954</td><td></td><td colspan="3">13/64 = 20%</td><td colspan="3">9/37 = 24%</td><td colspan="3">5/29 = 17%</td><td colspan="2">2/8 = 25%</td></tr>
<tr><td>Singer et al.</td><td>1956</td><td></td><td colspan="3">14%</td><td colspan="3">17%</td><td>21%</td><td colspan="4"></td></tr>
<tr><td>Crehange</td><td>1958</td><td></td><td>4/12=33%</td><td colspan="2">8/37/22%</td><td>7/33=21%</td><td colspan="2">6/16=38%</td><td>9/17=50%</td><td colspan="4"></td></tr>
<tr><td>Goddé (cit. from Crehange)</td><td>1958</td><td></td><td>10/33=30%</td><td colspan="2">15/54=24%</td><td>6/36=17%</td><td colspan="2">2/13=15%</td><td>4/19=21%</td><td colspan="4"></td></tr>
<tr><td rowspan="2">Koyama</td><td rowspan="2">1959</td><td>P</td><td colspan="3">9/23=39%</td><td colspan="3">17/66=26%</td><td colspan="2">16/50=32%</td><td>9/37=24%</td><td>3/10=30%</td><td>20/45=22%</td></tr>
<tr><td>M</td><td colspan="3">28/105=27%</td><td colspan="3">23/98=24%</td><td colspan="2">11/47=23%</td><td>5/13=39%</td><td>2/ 5</td><td>0/11</td></tr>
<tr><td rowspan="2">Motohashi and Kobayashi</td><td rowspan="2">1960</td><td>P</td><td colspan="3">3/17=18%</td><td colspan="3">7/30=23%</td><td colspan="2">5/18=28%</td><td>2/10=20%</td><td>4/10</td><td>3/ 9</td></tr>
<tr><td>M</td><td colspan="3">12/49=25%</td><td colspan="3">3/23=13%</td><td colspan="2">1/15= 7%</td><td>2/ 6</td><td>1/ 5</td><td>0/ 1</td></tr>
<tr><td>Kawakami</td><td>1963</td><td></td><td colspan="3">20/81=25%</td><td colspan="7">lesser numbers</td><td>14/87=16%</td></tr>
<tr><td rowspan="2">Kobayashi et al.</td><td rowspan="2">1964</td><td>P</td><td colspan="3">2/ 6=33%</td><td colspan="3">2/14=43%</td><td>3/12=25%</td><td>6/19=32%</td><td>1/ 5</td><td></td><td>4/11</td></tr>
<tr><td>M</td><td colspan="3">3/15=20%</td><td colspan="3">2/16=13%</td><td>1/ 6=17%</td><td>0/ 4</td><td>0/ 1</td><td></td><td>0/ 1</td></tr>
<tr><td>Jain and Gupta</td><td>1965</td><td></td><td colspan="3">9/30=30%</td><td colspan="3">15/47=30%</td><td colspan="3">21/53=40%</td><td colspan="2">2/11=18%</td></tr>
<tr><td rowspan="2">Pannarale</td><td rowspan="2">1966</td><td>P</td><td>0</td><td colspan="3">21%</td><td>32%</td><td>40%</td><td>42%</td><td>50%</td><td>51%</td><td colspan="2"></td></tr>
<tr><td>M</td><td>30%</td><td colspan="3">22%</td><td>28%</td><td>28%</td><td>21%</td><td>25%</td><td>22%</td><td colspan="2"></td></tr>
<tr><td>Santamarina</td><td>1969</td><td></td><td>3/21=14%</td><td colspan="5">27/145=19%</td><td>14/52=27%</td><td colspan="4">7/22=32%</td></tr>
<tr><td rowspan="2">v. Barsewisch</td><td rowspan="2">1972</td><td>P</td><td>0/ 1</td><td colspan="3">15/29=52%</td><td colspan="2">14/30=47% 7/11=64%</td><td>0/4</td><td colspan="2"></td><td>0/ 1</td><td></td></tr>
<tr><td>M</td><td>8/34=24%</td><td colspan="3">26/67=39%</td><td colspan="2">7/19=37% 1/ 3</td><td>0/1</td><td colspan="4"></td></tr>
<tr><td>Pommer</td><td>1972</td><td></td><td colspan="3">19/184=10%</td><td colspan="3">34/250=14%</td><td>21/141=15%</td><td colspan="4">17/93=18%</td></tr>
<tr><td>Krause</td><td>1974</td><td></td><td colspan="3">31/181=17%</td><td colspan="3">50/212=24%</td><td>15/ 73=21%</td><td colspan="4">5/22=23%</td></tr>
</table>

a P, primiparae; M, multiparae.

No significant tendency can be deduced from this table. With longer duration of labour, the incidence of retinal haemorrhage was found to be higher by McKeown (1941), Singer et al. (1956), Pannarale (1966) and Santamarina (1969). The opposite is seen in the figure of Kawakami et al. (1963). In all series, extreme values comprise a few cases only, so that valid conclusions cannot be drawn.

Furthermore, the duration of labour has decreased nowadays, which can be seen by comparing earlier auhtors with recent ones. In the I. Frauenklinik der Universität München the mean value for a delivery was 18 h in 1900 and has now been reduced to 6.7 h (Martius, 1971). The time in which half the births are completed has been reduced from 14 h to 6.2 h.

The report of Döring and Krauss (1967) on 7860 births at the I. Frauenklinik der Universität München between 1955 and 1962 shows a mortality for newborns of 0.33%. With a duration over 30 h, the mortality increased to 3.2%. With a second stage of labour of up to 14 min, mortality was 0.1%; between 15 and 29 min, 0.3%; between 30 and 49 min, 0.8%; with duration over 50 min, 1%.

With longer duration of the first stage of labour, mortality rises (Hickl, 1972). Very clearly, the incidence of asphyxia depends on the duration of the first and second stages of labour.

In our series of 200 spontaneous deliveries, there were 12 cases with a total duration of labour longer than 10 h and a single case with a duration of 24 h. The incidence of haemorrhages in these cases was not elevated, possibly because in these cases the second stage of labour did not exceed 30 min, except one case of 60 min. It is therefore desirable to consider the material not according to total duration of labour, but according to duration of first and second stages, respectively.

b) First Stage

The first stage of labour seems to have little influence on the incidence of retinal haemorrhage. It appears that several authors did not publish their figures because they did not find a correlation. Vincenti and Gavinelli (1969) report that all infants with haemorrhages were born after a first stage of labour of more than 8 h. But this does not indicate anything because all these infants were born after a second stage of labour of more than 1 h, which is more significant. The figures from the literature are given in Table 15.

c) Second Stage

Kauffman (1941) reports, without further details, that the incidence of haemorrhage increases with very short and very long second stages of labour. More data from the literature can be found in Table 16.

Considering discrepancies in the data, it is difficult to come to any conclusion. The author's observation of 71% haemorrhage where the second stage of labour exceeds 30 min points to a positive correlation. It seems clear that foetal compensation is sufficient in even a prolonged first stage of labour but not in a prolonged second stage. As a result a higher rate of hypoxia develops (Hickl and von Barsewisch, 1969). Giles (1960) and Panagiotou et al. (1968) stressed that very short second stages are correlated with a higher incidence of haemorrhage.

Table 15. First stage of labour and incidence of haemorrhages

<table>
<tr><td rowspan="2">Author, year</td><td rowspan="2">a</td><td colspan="24">Hours</td></tr>
<tr><td>1</td><td>2</td><td>3</td><td>4</td><td>5</td><td>6</td><td>7</td><td>8</td><td>9</td><td>10</td><td>11</td><td>12</td><td>13</td><td>14</td><td>15</td><td>16</td><td>17</td><td>18</td><td>19</td><td>20</td><td>21</td><td>22</td><td>23</td><td>24</td></tr>
<tr><td>Lomíčková and Otradovec, 1965</td><td></td><td colspan="3">12/68=39%</td><td colspan="3">31/125=25%</td><td colspan="6">56/180=31%</td><td colspan="11">26/61=33%</td><td colspan="1">8/15=54%</td></tr>
<tr><td rowspan="2">Takala and Sopanen 1967</td><td>P</td><td colspan="12">40%</td><td colspan="8">44%</td><td colspan="4">39%</td></tr>
<tr><td>M</td><td colspan="12">25%</td><td colspan="8">20%</td><td colspan="4">43%</td></tr>
<tr><td>Schlaeder et al., 1971</td><td></td><td colspan="12">25/182=14%</td><td colspan="12">4/15=27%</td></tr>
<tr><td rowspan="2">v, Barsewisch, 1972</td><td>P</td><td colspan="3">2/4</td><td colspan="3">17/33=52%</td><td colspan="3">13/28=46%</td><td colspan="3">4/9=44%</td><td colspan="12">0/2</td></tr>
<tr><td>M</td><td colspan="3">9/8=24%</td><td colspan="3">25/62=40%</td><td colspan="3">7/20=35%</td><td colspan="3">1/3</td><td colspan="12">0/1</td></tr>
</table>

a P, primiparae, M, multiparae.

Table 16. Second stage of labour and incidence of retinal haemorrhage

<table>
<tr><th rowspan="2">Author</th><th rowspan="2">Year</th><th rowspan="2">a</th><th colspan="10">Minutes</th></tr>
<tr><th>< 5</th><th>6–10</th><th>11–15</th><th>16–20</th><th>21–25</th><th>26–30</th><th>31–40</th><th>41–50</th><th>51–60</th><th>> 60</th></tr>
<tr><td>Franceschetti and Balavoine</td><td>1951</td><td></td><td colspan="3">37/100=37%</td><td colspan="4">17/ 57=30%</td><td colspan="3">22/62=35%</td></tr>
<tr><td>Lomíčková and Otradovec</td><td>1956</td><td></td><td colspan="3">54/226=24%</td><td colspan="4">32/104=31%</td><td colspan="2">34/104=33%</td><td></td></tr>
<tr><td>Crehange</td><td>1958</td><td></td><td colspan="2">7/43=16%</td><td colspan="2">11/ 28=39%</td><td colspan="2">8/ 22=36%</td><td colspan="3">8/ 20=40%</td><td></td></tr>
<tr><td rowspan="2">Takala and Sopanen</td><td rowspan="2">1967</td><td>P</td><td colspan="7">36%</td><td colspan="2">64%</td><td>50%</td></tr>
<tr><td>M</td><td colspan="7">24%</td><td colspan="2">40%</td><td></td></tr>
<tr><td rowspan="2">Takeda</td><td rowspan="2">1968</td><td>P</td><td colspan="7">21/109=19%</td><td colspan="2">21/ 58=36%</td><td>5/27=19%</td></tr>
<tr><td>M</td><td colspan="7">54/122=44%</td><td colspan="2">5/ 16=31%</td><td>0</td></tr>
<tr><td>Richter</td><td>1969</td><td></td><td>11%</td><td colspan="9">18%</td></tr>
<tr><td>Santamarina</td><td>1969</td><td></td><td colspan="7">36/208=17%</td><td colspan="3">11/36=31%</td></tr>
<tr><td>Loriaux and Toussaint</td><td>1971</td><td></td><td colspan="3">9/ 96= 9%</td><td colspan="7">6/17=35%</td></tr>
<tr><td>Schlaeder et al.</td><td>1971</td><td></td><td colspan="2">9/69=13%</td><td colspan="3">11/100=11%</td><td>4/ 16=25%</td><td>3/9</td><td>1/2</td><td colspan="2">1/1</td></tr>
<tr><td rowspan="2">v. Barsewisch</td><td rowspan="2">1972</td><td>P</td><td>3/ 5</td><td colspan="2">10/ 21=48%</td><td colspan="3">11/ 33=33%</td><td colspan="4">12/17=71%</td></tr>
<tr><td>M</td><td>8/41=20%</td><td colspan="2">29/ 70=41%</td><td colspan="3">5/ 11=45%</td><td colspan="4">0/ 1</td></tr>
<tr><td>Taleb Bandiab</td><td>1972</td><td></td><td>5/20=25%</td><td colspan="2">4/ 31=13%</td><td colspan="7">12/25=48%</td></tr>
<tr><td>Ciechanowska et al.</td><td>1974</td><td></td><td colspan="7">ca. 20%</td><td colspan="3">ca. 40%</td></tr>
<tr><td rowspan="2">Zisa et al.</td><td rowspan="2">1975</td><td>P</td><td>0/ 5</td><td colspan="5">29/223=13%</td><td>6/46=13%</td><td>1/9</td><td colspan="2"></td></tr>
<tr><td>M</td><td>2/34= 6%</td><td colspan="5">48/439=11%</td><td>1/19</td><td>0</td><td colspan="2"></td></tr>
</table>

a P, primiparae, M, multiparae.

As to the severity of haemorrhage in our material, no correlation could be found because the more severe haemorrhages were equally distributed in different groups

The perineal stage of labour is considered to be important by Jain and Gupta (1965): Head on the perineum for less than 15 min led to 29.2% haemorrhage; a perineal stage of labour of more than 15 min, to 75% haemorrhage.

d) Rupture of Foetal Membranes

Early rupture of foetal membranes has been considered the cause of a higher incidence of retinal haemorrhage (Kauffman, 1941; Jirman, 1947; Koyama, 1959; Neuweiler and Onwudiwe, 1967; Pommer, 1972, especially with primiparae; Puskás and Szabó, 1962, with a low value only). Lukaszewicz and Zaporowski (1969) found more severe retinal haemorrhage after early rupture of the membrane. No connection was seen by Stumpf and von Sicherer (1909), Cavrot et al. (1955), Motohashi and Kobayashi (1960) and Kawakami et al. (1963).

8. Drugs Administered During Labour

Vitamins and other drugs given to prevent or reduce the amount of haemorrhage will be discussed in Section D of this chapter. In the present section, pituitary preparations and anaesthetics administered during labour will be considered.

a) Pituitary Preparations

These have been related to a higher incidence of retinal haemorrhage. Again, it has to be considered that they would be administered in the case of a slowly progressing birth, so that foetal hypoxia may be involved. No correlation was found by Santamarina (1969). Other authors report a positive correlation, sometimes with series too small for a proper evaluation:

Motohashi and Kobayashi (1960): Control group = 16.7% haemorrhages
    With Spatym, 15 haemorrhages out of 35 cases = 41.2%
    With Atonin O, 5 haemorrhages out of 27 cases = 18.5%
Kawakami et al. (1963): General series = 19.5%
    With pituitary preparations = 32.35%
Sanchez-Ibanez et al. (1963): Normal group = 32.5%
    With pituitary preparations = 48.7%
Takeda (1968): Normal cases, 90 haemorrhages out of 379 cases = 23.7%
    With oxytocin, 51 haemorrhages out of 142 cases = 39.5%
Loriaux and Toussaint (1971): Without oxytocin, 11/103 = 11%
    With oxytocin, 6/32 = 19%
Author's series of 1972: Without pituitary preparations, 39/119 = 33%
    With pituitary preparations, 38/80 = 48%

A correlation seems to exist, though, as mentioned before, it is probably due more to foetal hypoxia leading to the administration of pituitary preparations than to the drugs administered.

b) Anaesthetics

Casanovas et al. (1959) and Takeda (1968) compared the cases of infants born with and without anaesthesia. Owing to the influence of anaesthetics on the coagulability of infantile blood (Sanford, 1926), a higher incidence of retinal haemorrhage might have ensued, but both authors could find no evidence of this. Zisa et al. (1975) found a higher rate of retinal haemorrhage after anaesthesia, possibly due to prologation of delivery. Without anaesthesia: primiparae 8/103 = 8%, multiparae 18/122 = 8%; with anaesthesia: primiparae 29/181 = 16%, multiparae 31/270 = 12%.

9. Summary

After spontaneous delivery from occipital presentation, about 1/3 of the newborn infants have retinal haemorrhages. A correlation of one side with left or right occipital presentation cannot be established.

Obstetric procedures reducing a prolonged second stage of labour, such as forceps delivery and vacuum extraction, are connected with a higher incidence of retinal haemorrhage by a factor of 1.5–2. It must be assumed that it is not so much the procedure itself but the condition necessitating its use that is responsible for the higher incidence of haemorrhage.

Breech presentation is connected with very few haemorrhages, and these seem to occur mainly if other obstetric complications are present at the same time. Caesarian section is also connected with fewer haemorrhages and, if these occur, it seems to be after attempted labour or after the onset of asphyxia.

Long duration of labour seems to increase the frequency of haemorrhage, especially a prolonged second stage. Pituitary preparations are associated with a higher frequency of haemorrhage but are administered only to reduce the length of a labour which would otherwise be prolonged.

Zusammenfassung

Nach Spontanentbindung aus Hinterhauptslage haben etwa 1/3 der Neugeborenen Netzhautblutungen. Eine Korrelation der Seitenbetonung zur rechten oder linken Hinterhauptslage findet sich nicht. Geburtshilfliche Eingriffe, die eine verlängerte Austreibungsperiode abkürzen, wie Zangenentbindung oder Vakuumextraktion sind mit einer um den Faktor 1,5 bis 2 erhöhten Blutungsrate korreliert. Es ist anzunehmen, daß weniger der Eingriff als solcher, als die Indikation für den Eingriff zur höheren Blutungsfrequenz führt. Bei Beckenendlagen treten wenige Blutungen auf, vorwiegend wohl, wenn andere geburtshilfliche Komplikationen mitspielen. Nach Kaiserschnitt werden Blutungen fast nur nach versuchter Spontangeburt oder eingetretener Asphyxie gefunden. Lange Geburtsdauer, speziell eine verlängerte Austreibungsperiode sind mit erhöhter Blutungsfrequenz korreliert. Hypophysenpräparate ebenfalls, jedoch wahrscheinlich über die verlängerte Geburtsdauer.

B. Maternal Factors

1. Parity

Stumpf and Sicherer (1909) found almost twice as many infants with retinal haemorrhage born to primiparous mothers. There are a considerable number of references (Table 17).

From this table, an inverse relation has been stated by Tsopelas and Charamis (1955), who tried to justify the result with a higher age for multiparous mothers, and by Falls and Jurow (1946) and Martinez and Grom (1969). No difference was found by Grassi and Musini (1950), Terado (1953), Yamanouchi (1959), Sanchez-Ibanez et al. (1963) and Wierhake (1971). Without publishing figures, other authors found no relation: Bachmann et al. (1968), Fung (1968), Baum and Bulpitt (1970). But most of the authors report a definite prevalence of haemorrhage in primiparous mothers. Without figures this is stated by Drozdowa (1951), Buchhalter and Schnecke (1967) and Cavrot (1956), who thought that especially those children of older primiparae were affected. Comparing the figures of the different authors in Table 17 the relation of perinatal haemorrhage of primiparae to that of multiparae is 3:2 or 5:4 (as in the largest series, Kauffman, 1941).

Mayer and Maria (1952) found more severe haemorrhages in a group with lower mean parity. In our series, this could not be confirmed, since the intense haemorrhages (groups 4 and 5) represent about 1/2 of the haemorrhages: primiparae: 76 cases, 36 haemorrhages, of which 16 were light (groups 2 and 3) and 20 severe (groups 4 and 5). Multiparae: 124 cases, 42 haemorrhages, among which 20 were light and 22 severe.

The higher incidence of retinal haemorrhage in children from primiparous mothers was attributed mainly to the rigidity of the birth canal. Unfortunately only a few data have been published about the duration of the second stage of labour. According to our observations, a correlation between a prolonged second stage of labour and primiparity has to be suspected. Among our 200 observations, there were 110 multiparae with a second stage of labour of less than 15 min (cf. Table 14). The incidence of retinal haemorrhage was 34%. A second stage of labour of more than 30 min was observed in only 1 multipara (in this case without haemorrhage). But there were 17 primiparae with a second stage of labour exceeding 30 min and, in this group, there were 71% haemorrhages. The figures published by Takala and Sopanen (1967) document the same tendency.

So it seems likely that the influence of parity is mainly due to a prolonged second stage of labour in primiparae. The publication of more exact figures on this would be desirable.

2. Age of Mother

Here the results are very controversial. References are collected in Table 18.

As in the most of the other tables, the extreme values are very small, so that percentages cannot be compared. There seems to be hardly any correlation. Searching for

Table 17. Parity and incidence of retinal haemorrhages

Author	Year	Primiparae	Multiparae
Stumpf and von Sicherer	1909	25/100 = 25%	12/ 100 = 12%
Ko	1925	36%	29%
Eades	1929	16/ 69 = 23%	8/ 69 = 12%
Sykes	1931	36/107 = 33%	38/ 205 = 18%
Edgerton	1934	138/315 = 44%	52/ 196 = 27%
Kauffman	1941	119/578 = 21%	278/1735 = 16%
McKeown	1941	126/244 = 52%	64/ 254 = 25%
Nakajima	1943	6/ 17 = 35%	3/ 18 = 17%
Falls and Jurow	1946	23%	52%
Belmonte-Gonzales	1947	22/ 62 = 36%	12/ 62 = 19%
Jirmán	1947	74%	40%
Grassi and Musini	1950	20/142 = 14%	22/ 158 = 14%
Millán and Beltrán	1950	18/ 83 = 22%	12/ 72 = 17%
Štefek	1951	22%	13%
Terado	1953	7/ 16 = 44%	8/ 19 = 42%
Nevinny-Stickel	1954	39/ 64 = 47%	17/ 60 = 28%
Tsópelas and Charamis	1955	78/ 18 = 21%	20/ 75 = 27%
Lomíčková and Otradovec	1956	90/266 = 43%	47/ 234 = 20%
Lemmingson and Stark	1957	42/123 = 34%	32/ 144 = 22%
Crehange	1958	20/ 46 = 44%	17/ 69 = 25%
Ishikawa	1959	16/ 55 = 30%	4/ 20 = 20%
Yamanouchi	1959	6/ 29 = 21%	11/ 49 = 22%
Giles	1960	9/ 10 = 90%	7/ 37 = 29%
Motohashi and Kobayashi	1960	24/ 96 = 25%	19/ 104 = 18%
Puskás and Szabó	1961	235/547 = 43%	134/ 397 = 24%
Brogi et al.	1962	69/383 = 15%	78/ 395 = 20%
Sanchez-Ibanez et al.	1963	35/103 = 34%	74/ 221 = 33%
Treit et al.	1964	38/194 = 20%	25/ 152 = 15%
Gajaria et al.	1965	10/ 29 = 34%	33/ 171 = 19%
Jain and Gupta	1965	22/ 60 = 37%	25/ 110 = 23%
Konstantopais	1965	82/ 15 = 18%	98/ 31 = 32%
Krebs and Jäger	1966	18%	13%
Pannarale	1966	70/210 = 33%	73/ 335 = 22%
Schenker and Gombos	1966	25%	under 17%
Maertens and Götz	1967	7/ 14 = 50%	20/ 73 = 27%
Neuweiler and Onwudiwe	1967	39%	29%
Panagiotou et al.	1967	173/555 = 31%	211/ 665 = 32%
de Freitas and Garcia	1968	6/ 20 = 30%	21/ 79 = 27%
Tranou-Sphalangakou	1968	29/ 64 = 45%	26/ 125 = 21%
Lukaszewicz and Zaporowski	1969	31%	26%
Martinez and Grom	1969	16/ 80 = 13%	6/ 42 = 14%
Richter	1969	24%	14%
Sezen	1970	81/406 = 20%	94/ 832 = 11%
Loriaux and Toussaint	1971	6/ 32 = 19%	9/ 105 = 9%
Schlaeder et al.	1971	9/ 46 = 20%	20/ 152 = 13%
Wierhake	1971	38%	37%
v. Barsewisch	1972	36/ 76 = 47%	42/ 125 = 34%
Neme et al.	1972	16/ 43 = 37%	26/ 146 = 18%
Pommer	1972	52/259 = 20%	39/ 409 = 10%
Taleb Bendiab	1972	14/ 26 = 54%	15/ 74 = 20%
Hoo	1973	6/ 17 = 35%	12/ 83 = 14%
Ciechanowska	1974	42%	15%
Ehlers et al.	1974	110/259 = 42%	47/ 141 = 33%
Krause et al.	1974	72/283 = 25%	29/ 217 = 13%
Zisa	1975	87/836 = 10%	50/ 492 = 10%

Table 18. Age of mother and incidence of retinal haemorrhages (retinal haemorrhages/cases = percent)

Author	Year	a	< 20 yr	21–25 yr	26–30 yr	31–35 yr	36–40 yr	> 40 yr
Lomíčková and Otradovec	1956	T	20/ 63 = 32%	93/333 = 28%			24/102 = 24%	0/2
		P		79/213 = 34%			11/ 35 = 32%	
		M		34/164 = 21%			13/ 70 = 19%	
Singer et al.	1956	P	22%	24%				50%
		T	22%	20%				24%
Koyama	1959	P	6/ 4 = 67%	31/127 = 24%	22/ 77 = 29%	6/ 17 = 35%	3/ 1 = 33%	0/1
		M		18/ 64 = 28%	36/141 = 26%	13/ 56 = 23%	0/10	2/8
Motohashi and Kobayashi	1960	P	1/ 8 = 13%	10/ 50 = 20%	11/ 29 = 38%	2/ 8	0/ 1	
		M		2/ 18 = 11%	13/ 64 = 20%	3/ 15 = 20%	1/ 7 = 14%	
Puskás and Szabó	1961	T	42/ 99 = 42%	132/348 = 38%	117/290 = 40%	59/139 = 42%	15/63 = 24%	4/5
Jain and Gupta	1965	T	2/ 14 = 14%	44/138 = 32%		0/ 12	2/ 6	
Konstantopais	1965	T	8/ 40 = 20%	10/ 52 = 19%	16/ 54 = 30%	7/ 22 = 32%	5/12 = 42%	
Pannarale	1966	T	24%	28%	26%	23%	27%	
Panagiotou et al.	1968	T	16/ 69 = 23%	99/455 = 22%		35/164 = 21%	15/57 = 26%	
v. Barsewisch	1972	P	12/ 26 = 46%	15/ 31 = 48%	6/ 15 = 40%	2/ 3	1/ 1	
		M	0/ 6	10/ 30	12/ 44 = 27%	12/ 32 = 38%	6/10	2/2
Krause et al.	1974	T	31/135 = 23%	48/208 = 23%	10/ 98 = 10%	9/ 46 = 20%	3/13	

a   T, total series; P, primiparae; M, multiparae.

an influential factor correlated with the age of the mother, we might find it to be the second stage of labour. In our series there were 26 primiparae under 20 years with a mean time for second stage of labour of 24 min, ranging from 5 to 62 min. A direct coordination of cases with haemorrhages and long second stages was not possible. The 6 multiparae under 20 years had a mean duration of second stage of labour of 6 min (2–15 min) and here no haemorrhages were observed.

The severity of haemorrhages was not found to be correlated with age.

3. Other Maternal Factors

Contracted pelvis is an item frequently discussed in the old literature (Schleich, 1884; Naumoff, 1890; Montalcini, 1897; Paul, 1900). Sometimes it is discussed in connection with forceps delivery (Powelett and Townes, 1948). It is obvious that prolonged delivery and obstetric procedures can influence the incidence of retinal haemorrhage. With the performing of caesarian section, contracted pelvis has become less important.

Lequeux (1911) discussed syphilis as a factor: 50% of infants from syphilitic mothers had haemorrhages, compared with only 10% in the control group. A positive correlation was found by Štefek (1951), Mayer and Maria (1952), Dolcet-Buxeres and Ferrer-Pi (1954) and Mao (1959). No correlation was found by Eades (1929), Kauffman (1941), Grassi and Musini (1950), Koyama (1959), Puskás and Szabó (1961), Pannarale (1966). Walsh (1969) believes that syphilis is not a causal factor but that it could indirectly influence the matter by causing the birth of more immature infants.

Other factors discussed are: high blood pressure (Casanovas et al., 1959); eclampsia (Drozdowa, 1951); toxicosis (Lemmingson and Stark, 1957; Ishikawa, 1959; Kawakami et al., 1963). Rhesus factor incompatibility has been discussed by Jarny (1947), Grassi and Musini (1950) and Tranou-Sphalangakou (1968). Arranging their figures in a more usual way and eliminating errors in their calculations, the author cannot confirm the positive correlation with rhesus incompatibility that they suspected.

4. Summary

Parity is of definite influence on the frequency of retinal haemorrhages. This influence is most likely due to a prolonged second stage of labour in primiparous mothers. The influence of the age of the mother remains very uncertain. A low incidence of retinal haemorrhage in young multiparae seems, possibly, to be due to a short second stage of labour.

Zusammenfassung

Die Parität beeinflußt die Blutungsfrequenz deutlich. Dieser Einfluß ist wahrscheinlich auf die verlängerte Austreibungsperiode bei Primiparae zurückzuführen. Unsicher ist der Einfluß des Alters der Mutter. Möglicherweise findet sich bei jungen Multiparae eine geringe Blutungsfrequenz wegen einer kurzen Austreibungsperiode.

C. Infantile Factors

1. Sex Distribution

The first authors to publish detailed material about perinatal retinal haemorrhage from the obstetric point of view, Stumpf and von Sicherer (1909), found an incidence of haemorrhage in boys of 23.6% and in girls of 18.1%. This correlation was considered to be the result of the larger cranial circumference in boys. But the result has not been confirmed by later authors (Table 19). This table is of particular interest, not because a true correlation with number of boys or girls affected can be established but as an example of how unreliable the figures are, based on case samplings that were too small. The random distribution must be treated with particular suspicion. Tables trying to evaluate more complicated subgroups should be looked upon still more critically.

Table 19. Sex distribution and incidence of retinal haemorrhages

Author	Year	Boys	Girls
Stumpf and v. Sicherer	1909	24%	18%
McKeown	1941	112/234 = 48%	98/264 = 37%
Millán and Beltrán	1950	21/ 80 = 26%	9/ 65 = 14%
Cavrot	1956	49/225 = 22%	35/196 = 18%
Lomíčková and Otradovec	1956	63/244 = 26%	74/156 = 29%
Koyama	1959	62/258 = 24%	71/252 = 28%
Mao	1959	12%	20%
Yamanouchi	1959	11/ 40 = 28%	6/ 38 = 16%
Motohashi and Kobayashi	1960	25/111 = 23%	18/ 89 = 20%
Kobayashi	1964	13/ 64 = 20%	11/ 94 = 23%
Konstantopais	1965	26/ 95 = 27%	20/ 87 = 23%
Pannarale	1966	26%	26%
Neuweiler and Onwudiwe	1967	33%	34%
Sachsenweger	1967	23%	25%
Panagiotou et al.	1968	97/380 = 26%	68/365 = 19%
v. Barsewisch	1972	42/109 = 39%	35/ 88 = 40%
Zgorzalewicz et al.	1975	7/ 47 = 15%	8/ 53 = 15% [a]
		28/ 73 = 38%	14/ 37 = 38% [b]

a Spontaneous delivery.
b Vacuum extraction.

2. Weight and Size of the Newborn

The mean birth weight was found to be slightly elevated in cases with perinatal retinal haemorrhage by Schleich (1884), Falls and Jurow (1946) and Millán and Beltrán (1950). The differences, though, are very small. Most other authors dealing with this item classified the children according to their birth weight and the result is given in Table 20.

Table 20. Birth weight and incidence of retinal haemorrhages

Author	Year	< 1500 g	1500–2000 g	2000–2500 g	2500–3000 g	3000–3500 g	3500–4000 g	> 4000 g
Stumpf and v. Sicherer	1909		1/ 2=50%	5/18=28%	11/ 47=23%	21/ 91=23%	3/ 31=10%	1/ 11= 9%
Sykes	1939		5/ 5		17/ 90=23%	25/ 95=26%	20/ 96=21%	7/ 26=26%
Štefek	1951		11%		17%		16%	17%
Dolcet and Ferrer	1954		3/15=20%		5/ 31=16%	15/ 52=29%	6/ 40=15%	
Tsópelas and Charamis	1955			1/ 7	16/82=20%		6/40=15%	
Cavrot	1956			17/57=30%		36/189=19%	23/134=17%	8/ 41=20%
Lomíčková and Otradovec	1956		5/17=30%		67/226=30%		58/232=25%	7/25=36%
Singer et al.	1956			11%	18%	19%	17%	12%
Casanovas	1959	0/ 9	7/56=13%	4/35=11%				
Koyama	1959	0/ 3	1/ 2	9/36=25%	51/178=29%	58/224=26%	14/ 67=21%	
Yamanouchi	1959		0/ 5	1/ 6	6/ 29=21%	9/ 27=33%	1/ 11= 9%	
Motohashi and Kobayashi	1960		0/ 1	2/13=15%	13/ 60=22%	20/ 94=21%	7/ 29=24%	
Puskás and Szabó	1961			15/40=38%	125/304=41%	145/366=40%	78/192=41%	6/ 31=19%
Grigera	1964					19%		31%
Kawakami et al.	1964			3/30=10%	29/155=19%	45/213=21%	13/ 64=20%	2/ 9=22%
Kobayashi et al.	1964	0/ 1	0/ 1	4/11	8/ 30=27%	12/ 61=20%	1/12	
Treit et al.	1964		4/21=19%		16/ 80=20%	25/167=15%	11/ 64=17%	5/ 14=36%
Gajaria et al.	1965				28/123=23%	13/ 66=20%	2/ 10	0/ 1
Konstantopais	1965		5/15=33%		3/ 42= 7%	20/ 83=24%	12/ 32=38%	6/ 10
Moulène	1965		10/10	6/28=21%		1/ 32= 3%	14/25=56%	
Paufique et al.	1965					33%		58%
Krebs and Jäger	1966					< 20%		30–40%
Panagiotou et al.	1968		8/29=28%		34/147=23%	57/293=19%	56/240=23%	10/ 36=28%
Takeda	1968		2/ 7=29%		50/167=30%	66/250=26%	22/ 86=26%	1/ 11= 9%
Richter	1969		/15= 7%			/991=18%		/100=22%
Santamarina	1969		0/ 5		6/ 30=20%	39/178=22%		6/ 42=14%

<table>
<tr><td>Tranou-Sphalangakou</td><td>1969</td><td colspan="3"></td><td>24/ 64=35%</td><td>43/142=30%</td><td>35/121=21%</td><td></td></tr>
<tr><td>Loriaux and Toussaint</td><td>1971</td><td colspan="3">1/18</td><td>6/ 36=17%</td><td>19/ 85=22%</td><td>15/ 60=25%</td><td>3/ 12=17%</td></tr>
<tr><td>Schlaeder et al.</td><td>1971</td><td colspan="3">6/41=15%</td><td></td><td colspan="2">19/140=14%</td><td>4/ 17=24%</td></tr>
<tr><td>Szirmák</td><td>1971</td><td>2/32</td><td>3/57= 5%</td><td>11/60=18%</td><td>6/ 62=10%</td><td colspan="2">10/ 76=13%</td><td>1/ 12</td></tr>
<tr><td>Wierhake</td><td>1971</td><td colspan="3"></td><td>30%</td><td colspan="2">38%</td><td>54%</td></tr>
<tr><td>v. Barsewisch</td><td>1972</td><td colspan="2"></td><td>1/ 4</td><td>13/ 32=41%</td><td>30/ 78=38%</td><td>28/ 69=41%</td><td>6/ 16=38%</td></tr>
<tr><td>Pommer</td><td>1972</td><td colspan="3">3/44= 7%</td><td>15/140=11%</td><td>33/271=12%</td><td>38/175=16%</td><td>12/ 38=32%</td></tr>
<tr><td>Taleb Bendiab</td><td>1972</td><td colspan="3">4/11=36%</td><td>8/ 41=20%</td><td colspan="2">17/ 48=35%</td><td></td></tr>
<tr><td>Krause</td><td>1974</td><td colspan="3"></td><td>23/ 98=23%</td><td>44/239=18%</td><td>31/136=23%</td><td>3/ 27=11%</td></tr>
<tr><td>Zisa</td><td>1975</td><td colspan="3">P [a]</td><td>6/ 31=19%</td><td colspan="2">28/241=12%</td><td>0/ 12</td></tr>
<tr><td></td><td></td><td colspan="3">M</td><td>3/ 64= 5%</td><td colspan="2">41/370=11%</td><td>6/ 58=10%</td></tr>
</table>

a P, primiparae; M, multiparae.

Our observation is that the incidence of haemorrhage is fairly equally distributed between the weight groups of 2500–4000 g. There were no immature infants in our series; the four with a birth weight between 2300 and 2500 g were mature. The result deducible from Table 20 is that the average number of haemorrhages is also presented in the larger weight groups, between 3000 and 4000 g. Beyond these weight groups, again the extremes of the table comprise very small numbers and the percentage of haemorrhages becomes very unreliable. Some authors try to stress a tendency by classifying the material into two groups only. The classification according to the usual five or six weight groups might also have indicated no significant tendency. Without publishing figures, the following authors did not find birth weight to be influential: Sopanen (1966), Sachsenweger (1967), Buchhalter and Schnecke (1968), Fung et al. (1968), Takeda (1968), Weiden (1970).

Millán and Beltrán (1950) found a slight difference in length of the body between the group with haemorrhages (average 50.43 cm) and the one without haemorrhages (average 49.6 cm). Weiden (1970) found no relation, and nor did we (Table 21).

Table 21. Size of infant and incidence of retinal haemorrhages

Body length (cm)	45	46	47	48	49	50	51	52	53	54	55	56
Cases	1	1	5	12	25	36	28	35	23	16	7	5
Haemorrhages	0	0	0	5	7	17	12	13	9	4	4	0

3. Cranial Circumference

Stumpf and von Sicherer (1909) thought that retinal haemorrhages could be influenced by the size of the foetal head. Their main figures are:

Suboccipito-bregmatic circumference:
normal 31.7 cm, with haemorrhages 32.2 cm
Fronto-occipital circumference:
normal 33.2–33.8 cm, with haemorrhages 34.31 cm

Further details and the percentage of haemorrhages found:

Medium width of fontanels and sutures: 16.1%
Hard cranium: 27.4%
Soft cranium: 14.4%
Defects in the ossification: 9%

Since that publication, the details concerning the foetal cranium have never been published with the same accuracy. Some figures were published by Tranou-Sphalangakou. She also found a slightly higher incidence of haemorrhage with larger crania. The author's material is compared with these results in Table 22. Again the numbers at the extremes are much too small for any conclusion to be drawn. Baum and Bulpitt (1970) found no positive correlation.

Table 22. Cranial circumference and incidence of retinal haemorrhages

Author, year	Cranial circumference (cm)							
	31	32	33	34	35	36	37	38
Tranou-Sphalan-gakou, 1968	0/7	16/59 = 27.5%			22/73 = 30%		4/10	
v. Barsewisch, 1972	0/1	2/8	13/30 = 43%	22/61 = 36%	23/51 = 45%	14/30 = 47%	1/9	2/4

A case of hydrocephalus with retinal haemorrhage was reported by Seefelder (1907). Belmonte-Gonzales (1947) tried to measure the pressure of the fontanels with a modified Schiötz tonometer. There were no clear results, and no relationship to intracranial haemorrhages could be found. He found the diameter of the fotanels to be influential.

4. Period of Gestation; Immaturity

The frequency of retinal haemorrhage in immature infants has been discussed many times in the literature. Because of the possible relationship to intracranial haemorrhage, causing the high mortality in these infants, it was hoped to find the two types of haemorrhage correlated. The comparatively well-visible retinal haemorrhages would have been a welcome indicator for intracranial bleeding of the foetus.

A considerable number of papers deal with the histologic findings of retinal haemorrhages in immature infants. Naumoff (1890) found no haemorrhages in 22 cases; Jacobs (1928), 2 cases with haemorrhages among four immature infants. More investigation was done after 1950, when retinal haemorrhage was seen in connection with retrolental fibroplasia. This disorder fully develops weeks after birth, so that no data on perinatal haemorrhage can be found in some of the series (Dixon and Paul, 1951; Laupus and Busquet, 1951; Busquet and Laupus, 1953). To study the process in the very early stages Reese et al. (1962) examined 282 (?) eyes of immature infants who weighed more than 300 g and found 72 (25%) retinal haemorrhages. Ten percent of the haemorrhages were located at the ora serrata. Ward (1954) found 39% haemorrhages among 41 infants who had died within the first week; Yoshioka (1954) found haemorrhages in 10 of 14 eyes; Calmettes et al. (1966) reported 1 case of haemorrhage among 5 infants who had lived less than 1 day. All these histologic investigations, dealing mainly with the question of retrolental fibroplasia, did not reveal any new details concerning the histology of perinatal haemorrhage.

The clinical investigations with early fundus examination are not very helpful, either, for discussing perinatal haemorrhage. There are considerable difficulties in making the fundus of the premature newborn visible. Tyner (1952) reports about unclear media in some cases and about an opaque film on the cornea (Jochmus, 1968; Honegger, 1969). The tunica vasculosa lentis, still present in immature infants prior to the 32nd week, makes fundus photographs impossible (Baum, 1971). The results concerning the fundus examinations of immature infants are collated in Table 23.

Table 23. Retinal haemorrhages in immature infants, clinical series

Author	Year	Immature infants	Mature infants	Examination date; remarks
Paul	1900	?/ 17=40%	20%	Mainly 1st to 3rd day. 3 under 200 g without haemorrhages
Stumpf and von Sicherer	1909	11/ 34=32%	32/ 166=19%	1st day
Kauffman	1941	3/ 23=13%	397/2331=17%	1st to 3rd day
Tyner	1952	10/200= 5%		Examination date?
Dorello and Poli	1953	0/ 45		Examination date 10th to 30th day
Ferreira	1955	0/ 39		Only 5 on 1st day, others up to 15th day
Kästner	1957	19/129=15%		2nd to 3rd week, haem. without retrolental fibroplasia
Casanovas et al.	1959	11/ 83=13%		Within 1st week
Yamanouchi	1959	1/ 5	16/ 73=22%	Examination date?
Motohashi and Kobayashi	1960	2/ 11	34/ 162=21%	1st day
Puskás and Szabó	1961	15/ 40=38%	39%	1st day
Brogi et al.	1962	2/ 28= 7%	236/1560=15%	1st and 2nd day
Hosaka	1963	8/ 60=22%	19%	36 on 1st day
Makayama	1963	11/ 42=26%		Up to 4th day
Fontaine	1971	15—20%		No details
Szirmák	1971	16/150=11%	17/ 150=11%	Immature on 2nd day, mature on 1st day

In most of the cases the examination date is too late for observing perinatal haemorrhage. But even papers with earlier examinations and those comparing mature and immature infants do not offer uniform observations. A higher incidence of retinal haemorrhage in immature children was observed mainly by early authors, e.g. Sykes (1931) found bilateral haemorrhaging in the five children with a birth weight under 2500 g in his series. The more recent publications all report a lower incidence of perinatal retinal haemorrhage in immature infants. The overall incidence might be 15%—20%, as compared to 30%—40% in mature infants. Therefore, the figures of Joppich and Schulte (1968), of 50%—60%, or Douglas (1969), of 90% must be based on misunderstood quotations from early authors.

It is conceivable that two different factors influence the incidence of haemorrhage in immature infants: The smaller cranial circumference might reduce the trauma of delivery. On the other hand, the immaturity of retinal vessels might lead to greater vulnerability. Heath (1950) found retinal haemorrhages more frequently in immature children born relatively close to the end of the gestation period. Nakayama (1963) found no correlation with the different weight groups of immature infants. The period of gestation is mentioned by a few authors; the results are given in Table 24.

All figures, collected here, including our material, are too small for any tendency to be deduced from them.

Table 24. Period of gestation and incidence of retinal haemorrhages

<table>
<tr><td rowspan="2">Author</td><td rowspan="2">Year</td><td colspan="8">Weeks</td></tr>
<tr><td>36</td><td>37</td><td>38</td><td>39</td><td>40</td><td>41</td><td>42</td><td>43</td></tr>
<tr><td>Terado</td><td>1953</td><td>1/3</td><td colspan="3">6/17 = 35%</td><td colspan="4">8/15 = 53%</td></tr>
<tr><td>Pannarale</td><td>1966</td><td colspan="4">133/495 = 27%</td><td colspan="4">6/27 = 22%</td></tr>
<tr><td>Takeda</td><td>1968</td><td colspan="2">10/20 = 50%</td><td colspan="4">118/474 = 25%</td><td colspan="2">13/27 = 49%</td></tr>
<tr><td>v. Barsewisch</td><td>1972</td><td>2/2</td><td>4/16 = 25%</td><td>7/19 = 37%</td><td>20/30 = 66%</td><td>14/68 = 35%</td><td>16/37 = 43%</td><td>1/5</td><td>0/2</td></tr>
</table>

5. Asphyxia

Several authors have discussed the role of asphyxia, although its definition in the material is not uniform. In some cases intrauterine asphyxia is meant. The results are collated in Table 25.

Table 25. Asphyxia and incidence of retinal haemorrhages

Author	Year	Infants with asphyxia	Infants without asphyxia	Total series
Stumpf and v. Sicherer	1909	6/18 = 33%	36/182 = 20%	
McKeown	1941	12/48 = 25%	198/450 = 44%	
Millán and Beltrán	1950	14/34 = 41%	16/121 = 13%	
Dolcet and Ferrer	1954	5/12 = 42%	27/212 = 13%	
Tsópelas and Charamis	1955	5/ 9 = 56%		32/135 = 23%
Lomíčková and Otradovec	1956	54/92 = 59%	130/308 = 42%	
Lemmingson and Stark	1957	5/10 = 50%		74/264 = 28%
Koyama	1959	12/39 = 31%	121/471 = 26%	
Motohashi and Kobayashi	1960	43/ 9 = 33%	40/191 = 21%	
Puskás and Szabó	1961	7/12 = 51%		369/944 = 39%
Kawakami et al.	1963	6/25 = 24%		92/771 = 20%
Kobayashi	1964	3/10 = 30%	21/103 = 20%	
Treit et al.	1964	3/ 9 = 33%		42/255 = 17%
Jain and Gupta	1965	3/21 = 14%		47/170 = 28%
Pannarale	1966	38%		143/550 = 26%
Panagiotou et al.	1968	42/65 = 64%		165/745 = 22%
Stafanini et al.	1968	14/20 = 70% [a]	8/ 26 = 31%	
Richter	1969	18/82 = 22%	165/967 = 17%	
Santamarina	1969	10/20 = 50%		51/250 = 20%
Wierhake	1971	8/15 = 53%	100/263 = 38%	

a   Vacuum extraction.

Most of the authors confirm a higher incidence of perinatal retinal haemorrhage in asphyctic infants. A lower rate was found only by Eades (1927), Baum and Bulpitt (1970, mainly immature children) and Ehlers et al. (1974). The author's result is given according to the Apgar score, together with the few other comparable data from the literature (Table 26). Here a tendency seems to be clear: Children with a lower Apgar score tend to have a higher incidence of retinal haemorrhage. In our series the scores were mainly Apgar 8 and 9, and in this group there were 41% haemorrhages, the average value of the whole series. Of 22 children with an Apgar score of 7 and less, 11 were found to have haemorrhages.

The positive correlation of asphyxia with a higher incidence of retinal haemorrhage is of importance. Asphyxia occurs in prolonged labour and requires obstetric intervention. These latter are connected with a higher incidence of haemorrhage. Hypoxia can cause vessel dilatation and thus furnish one pathogenetic factor of retinal haemorrhage. Krause et al. (1974) went so far as to evaluate the effect of continuous electronic monitoring of the birth by observing the frequency of hypoxia-influenced retinal haemorrhage.

Table 26. Apgar score and incidence of retinal haemorrhages

<table>
<thead>
<tr><th>Author</th><th>Year</th><th>< 6</th><th>6</th><th>7</th><th>8</th><th>9</th><th>10</th></tr>
</thead>
<tbody>
<tr><td>Neuweiler and Onwudiwe</td><td>1967</td><td colspan="3">40%</td><td colspan="3">35%</td></tr>
<tr><td>Takeda</td><td>1968</td><td colspan="3">13/36=36%</td><td colspan="3">128/516=25%</td></tr>
<tr><td>Santamarina</td><td>1969</td><td colspan="4">21/49=43%</td><td colspan="2">29/210=14%</td></tr>
<tr><td>Schlaeder et al.</td><td>1971</td><td colspan="4">4/ 8=50%</td><td colspan="2">25/189=13%</td></tr>
<tr><td>v. Barsewisch</td><td>1972</td><td colspan="3">11/22=50%</td><td colspan="2">64/157=41%</td><td>3/20=15%</td></tr>
<tr><td>Taleb Bendiab</td><td>1972</td><td>5/5=100%</td><td colspan="2">7/15=47%</td><td colspan="3">17/ 80=21%</td></tr>
<tr><td>Bergen and Margolis</td><td>1976</td><td colspan="2">6/12=50%</td><td colspan="2">9/25=33%</td><td colspan="2">20/61=33%</td></tr>
</tbody>
</table>

6. Other Infantile Factors

Intraocular pressure has also been taken into consideration. Dolcet-Buxeres and Ferrer-Pi (1954) reported values of 48–56 mm Hg in newborn infants. This is very much in contradiction to the general opinion. Casanovas et al. (1959) report an intraocular pressure between 15 and 16 mm Hg. Differences in intraocular pressure between groups with or without retinal haemorrhage were not found.

7. Summary

Among the data collected on newborn infants, sex distribution and cranial circumference seem to be of no influence. Tables concerning this material must be regarded as typical examples of how unreliable evaluations are concerning extreme values in each series, which contain but a few figures.

Immaturity seems to be correlated to a lower incidence of perinatal retinal haemorrhage; the incidence in more recent observations is about 20%.

Asphyxia, especially if evaluated with the Apgar score, is correlated to a certain extent with a higher incidence of retinal haemorrhage. This is of fundamental interest because vessel dilatation, caused by asphyxia, represents one factor in the pathogenesis of vessel ruptures.

Zusammenfassung

Von den kindlichen Faktoren scheint die Geschlechtsverteilung und der Schädelumfang auf die Blutungsfrequenz keinen Einfluß zu haben. Das Geburtsgewicht hat höchstens einen geringen Einfluß. Tabellen, die dieses Material aufschließen, sind typische Beispiele für die Unzuverlässigkeit der verglichenen Serien, an deren Extrempunkten jeweils zu wenig Fälle untersucht wurden.

Frühgeburt scheint mit einer geringeren Blutungsfrequenz korreliert zu sein, in neueren Arbeiten liegt die Zahl bei 20%. Asphyxie, speziell nach dem Apgar-Wert beurteilt, ist zu einem gewissen Grad mit höherer Blutungsneigung gekoppelt. Dies ist von prinzipiellem Interesse, weil die durch Asphyxie hervorgerufene Gefäßdilatation einen Faktor in der Pathogenese von Gefäßrupturen darstellt.

D. Haemorrhagic Disease of the Newborn: Attempted Treatment

Hugo Ehrenfest discussed haemorrhagic diathesis as an underlying factor in retinal haemorrhage of the newborn in his inportant book *Birth Injuries of the Child* (1922). Since then, several authors have studied the haematologic aspect and some have attempted medical treatment of retinal haemorrhage.

1. Haemorrhagic Diathesis

True haemorrhagic diathesis of the newborn has an incidence of 1/2500, according to a 10 years' observation by Sanford et al. (1942). Kauffman found two cases among 3381 children. Of these one had retinal haemorrhages; the other, after a breech presentation, had none. This rare disease certainly plays no important part in the discussion of perinatal retinal haemorrhages.

Planten and v.d. Schaaf (1971) tried, without success, to correlate frequency of retinal haemorrhaging with the results of occult blood-tests. Icterus gravis is correlated with haemorrhages according to Kauffman (1941), whereas Pannarale (1966) found no correlation. Reduced viscosity of the blood is discussed as a causative factor by Candian (1949) and Baum and Bulpitt (1970), whereas Sachsenweger (1967) thinks it is not influential.

2. Prothrombin Time and Vitamin K

There are many significant differences between haematologic values of the adult and the newborn infant. Lucas et al. (1921) found a longer coagulation time and a reduced amount of prothrombin, but no prolongation of bleeding time in infants. Sanford et al. (1942) studied the level of prothrombin within the first days of life with Quick's method. The Quick test yielded 80% directly after birth, dropped to 20% at the 3rd day, and then rose to a value of 70% at the 7th—10th day. Similar results were found by Pray et al. (1941). Falls and Jurow (1946) demonstrated that administration of vitamin K to mothers prior to or during labour reduced this drop. Results of studies correlating prothrombin time with perinatal retinal haemorrhage are controversial (Grassi and Musini, 1950; Brogi et al., 1962; Paufique et al., 1965; Sezen, 1970).

Assuming that retinal haemorrhage is an important indicator of intracranial haemorrhage, some authors administered vitamin K as a prophylactic treatment. Maumenee et al. (1941) called the retina a more reliable indicator of haemorrhagic tendency than the cerebrospinal fluid or occult blood. Treating mothers with vitamin K during labour, they found a reduction in incidence of retinal haemorrhage from 25% to 15%. In 50 cases treated 4 days prior to birth only 4% haemorrhaging occurred. Since their fundus examinations were carried out up to the 5th day, we must regard their figures critically. But the authors were very positive: "The administration of vitamin K to mothers prior to the onset of labour almost entirely eliminates retinal haemorrhage in their infants." A positive effect was also seen by Pray et al. (1941), but with examamination dates as late as the 10th day. Other positive opinions were published by Wille (1946) and Terado (1953).

Falls and Jurow raised the level of prothrombin within the first days by administration of vitamin K. They did not, however, find a reduced incidence of retinal haemorrhage. Their explanation is that these haemorrhages occur during birth and not during the time when the level of prothrombin is reduced. No effect was found by Belmonte-Gonzales (1947), Yohitda et al. (1961), and after administration of vitamins B, C, and K by Mao (1959).

Kauffman (1958) had the broadest experience when he reported on 10,925 children. From 1941 to 1947 vitamin K had been applied as prophylaxis. Kauffman did not find a reduction in the number of retinal haemorrhages. The treatment was stopped when phlebitis was more frequently observed in the mothers. Sanford et al. (1942) had already doubted that raising the postnatal prothrombin level is a desirable effect. Some authors (Powelett and Townes, 1948; Grassi and Musini, 1950; Pontorieri and de Concillis, 1959) having administered vitamin K after birth (!), admit that no influence on retinal haemorrhages could have been expected.

The clotting time in the newborn has been studied by a few authors (Jacobs, 1924). Kozuhowska (1954) reports on three children with pathologic clotting times and extensive retinal haemorrhages, two of which increased postnatally! Tranou-Sphalangakou (1968) found 28% haemorrhages with a Quick test over 40% and a thrombofax test under 100 s (normal values) and 50% haemorrhages with a Quick test under 40% and a thrombofax test over 100 s (pathologic values). Künzer (1964) surveyed the physiology of coagulation in the newborn. Besides the activity of prothrombin, the amounts of fibrinogen and factors V, VII, VIII, IX and X are all reduced, and only gradulally gain the values typical for the adult. He denied that these differing laboratory results indicate pathologic coagulation conditions. "The physiology of the coagulation of the newborn appears to me an admonishing example for a longstanding misinterpretation of experimental results." He calls vitamin-K prophylaxis a fatal error, since it caused haemolysis and nuclear icterus in immature infants. That it caused phlebitis in mothers was mentioned before.

3. Capillary Resistance and Vitamin Prophylaxis

The capillary resistance in the newborn was found elevated in mature infants and reduced in immature ones by Minkowski (1949). Comparative examinations by Digonnet et al. (1952) with the capillary manometer of Lavollay produced less clear results. A relation to retinal haemorrhage has been postulated by some authors (Kozuhowska,

1954; Papousek, 1954, examining the material of Lomíčková and Otradovec, 1956; Tranou-Sphalangakou, 1968).

Assuming that capillary resistance – important for intracranial haemorrhage, especially in immature infants – could be influenced and possibly tested by fundus examinations, some authors adminstered drugs containing vitamins, with the following results:

Minkowski (1949): "Anti-fragilité vasculaire" = ascorbic acid, P-substances and vitamin E: 90 children without retinal haemorrhage (examination date?)

Mayer and Maria (1952): 50 mg vitamin K, 50 mg vitamin E, 10 mg vitamin P, 4 weeks prior to delivery: reduction of retinal haemorrhage from 36% to 22%

Cavrot et al. (1955): Vitamin C, vitamin E, rutin, hesperidin and vitamin K, 8 weeks prior to delivery: reduction of haemorrhage from 34% to 7%

Cavrot (1956): With the same substances: untreated 29.5%, treated 10.7% haemorrhage

Koyama (1959): Testing the preparation Hesna (Takeda Ltd./Osaka, Japan), a drug specifically produced and marketed for prophylaxis of perinatal retinal haemorrhage and consisting of: methylhesperidin 30 mg, rutin 20 mg, ascorbic acid 50 mg, adrenochromomonosemicarbazon 1 mg, vitamin K_1 0.5 mg, administered three times per day 10 days prior to delivery: reduction of retinal haemorrhage from 26% to 12%.

It should not be overlooked that mothers receiving vitamin or other prophylactic treatment prior to delivery constitute a selected group and may thereby entail fewer obstetric complications.

Hungarian authors found seasonal differences in the frequency of haemorrhage (Kerpel-Fronius, 1946; Puskás and Szabó, 1961). During winter and spring they found more haemorrhages and related this to a relative deficiency in vitamins. Reviewing our material according to seasons, the author found a random distribution.

Veinbaum (1967) believed that he could shorten the resorption time of retinal haemorrhages using vitamin K, a combination therapy of potassium and autoinoculations of blood. He simply compared his results with those in the literature (!) and had no control group.

4. Fibrinolysis and Fibrinolysis Inhibitors

According to Bleyl and Büsing (1970) intrauterine asphyxia causes hypercoagulability and a consumption of coagulation factors. This is not in accordance with the opinion of Ludwig (1968), who found intravasal fibrinolysis or fibrninogenolysis in the umbilical blood of newborns in asphyctic shock. Experimentally, he could prevent cerebral diapedesis haemorrhaging in rabbits by injection of a fibrinolysis inhibitor (epsilon-aminocaproic acid, a kallikrein-trypsin inactivator). It was then hoped the sequelae of perinatal shock could be prevented by an antenatal medical prophylaxis. To test the haemorrhage-preventing effect in the newborn, the fundus was examined. The results have been published (Hickl et al., 1970; Hickl, 1970; von Barsewisch and Hickl, 1971), but unfortunately cannot serve as an orientation: Without fibrinolysis inhibitor 46 out of 105 children had haemorrhages (44%); with fibrinolysis inhibitor, 48 out of 102 (47%). There were more severe haemorrhages with the fibrinolysis inhibitor: 36/81 eyes

(44%), as compared to the untreated series, which had 16/71 eyes (23%). The small group of vacuum extractions showed a different tendency: without fibrinolysis-inhibitor, 7/11 children (64%); with treatment, 14/32 children (44%). As in many other series, the figures seem too small for a proper evaluation. A significant influence of the fibrinolysis inhibitor could, at least, not be detected in these haemorrhages, caused by vessel ruptures, due to specific circulatory conditions during birth. This need not indicate, however, that postnatal intracranial haemorrhage by diapedesis, especially in immature infants, cannot be influenced by this prophylactic treatment.

Evsyukova and Reinish correlated spontaneous activity of fibrinolysis, influenced by time of ligation of the umbilical cord, with incidence of retinal haemorrhage. In 14 newborns, the cord was ligated immediately after birth: Fibrinolysis was positive in 2 infants (14%), and no haemorrhage was seen; in another 14 children, the ligation was performed after 120 s, causing spontaneous fibrinolysis activity in 11 cases (80%) and retinal haemorrhage in 7 (50%).

5. Summary

There seems to be a very limited influence of coagulation factors on the incidence of perinatal retinal haemorrhage. A prophylactic treatment of the mother with vitamin K before the birth or during labour may reduce the physiologic decrease in the prothrombin level in the newborn. This effect seems to be undesirable and even caused phlebitis in some mothers.

Positive results have been reported by administering vitamin preparations to elevate the capillary resistance in the newborn.

In one of our series, the influence of a fibrinolysis inhibitor on the incidence of retinal haemorrhage was tested. There seems to be no influence on the retinal haemorrhage, but this is no reliable indicator of the possible influence on intracranial diapedesis haemorrhaging.

Zusammenfassung

Ein sehr begrenzter Einfluß der Koagulationsfaktoren auf perinatale Netzhautblutungen kann vorliegen. Eine prophylaktische Vitamin-K-Behandlung der Mutter vor oder während der Entbindung kann den physiologischen Abfall des Prothrombinspiegels beim Neugeborenen verringern. Dieser Effekt erscheint überflüssig und hat außerdem bei den Müttern Phlebitis hervorgerufen.

Über positive Ergebnisse wurde berichtet bei Vitamin-Präparaten, die die Kapillarresistenz heraufsetzen. In einer eigenen Serie wurde der Einfluß eines Fibrinolyse-Hemmers auf die Häufigkeit der Netzhautblutungen untersucht. Dieser scheint keinen Einfluß auf die Häufigkeit der Netzhautblutungen zu haben, diese sind andererseits jedoch kein zuverlässiger Indikator für die mögliche Beeinflussung intracranieller Diapedeseblutungen.

E. Comparable Retinal Haemorrhages of Other Origin

Perinatal retinal haemorrhages have quite unjustifiably been studied by most authors as an isolated phenomenon. There are other related types of retinal haemorrhage which are worthwhile studying for a better understanding of the perinatal type. In addition the study of these is also useful for interpreting funduscopic and histologic detail of perinatal haemorrhages. For their pathogenesis, it is of interest that similar extravasations occur in disorders due to elevated pressure of the central retinal vein, i.e. venous occlusion, intracranial haemorrhage and trauma. The resulting haemorrhages are very similar to perinatal haemorrhages, although these latter are outstanding in that their time of onset is well defined.

1. Retinal Venous Occlusion

With early and, especially, with incomplete cases of retinal venous occlusion, the fresh state of retinal haemorrhage can be studied. Figure 60 demonstrates how similar the types of haemorrhages are. Haemorrhages of the nerve fibre layer, with typical flame-shaped appearance and central white thrombus, are visible. Typical granular haemorrhages of the internal granular layer are demonstrated in Figure 61. Naturally, with the long course of the circulatory disorder, these haemorrhages become less distinct and develop an amorphus appearance. In the newborn, the factors causing haemorrhage are different from these and act for a very short time only, and immediately after birth resorption begins.

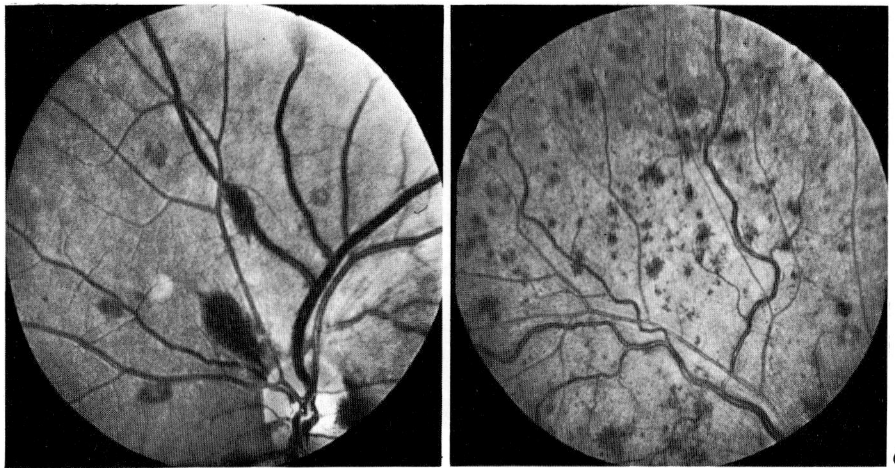

60   61

Fig. 60. 32-year-old patient with incomplete retinal vein occlusion. Dispersed haemorrhages of internal granular layer and typical flame-shaped haemorrhages of nerve fibre layer, with white centre, some of them passing over disc border

Fig. 61. 27-year-old patient with fresh central retinal vein occlusion. Multiple haemorrhages have typical granular structure and dendritic borders and can be clearly defined as belonging to granular layer

2. Intracranial Haemorrhage and Elevation of Cerebrospinal Fluid Pressure

Of all types of retinal haemorrhages, those caused by subarachnoid haemorrhage are most similar to the perinatal type. They occur in different retinal layers and can extend to the subretinal and preretinal spaces [cf. Doggarts (1950): subhyaloid haemorrhage, with blood cells collecting at the inferior margin].

According to the author's clinical examinations, all types of haemorrhages seen in the newborn can be found in cases of subarachnoid haemorrhage: Linear and flame-shaped haemorrhages of the nerve fibre layer, granular haemorrhages of the internal granular layer and submembranacious haemorrhages. Clinical descriptions in the literature very often lack the knowledge of histologic detail and thus are less reliable. Many authors have properly described the haemorrhages confined to the nerve fibre layer. Aust et al. (1967) and Schmidt and Trojan (1970) also describe cockade-shaped haemorrhages, which certainly represent the granular type. Pale centres of haemorrhages were described by Phelps (1971) but remained unexplained. Submembranacious haemorrhages are illustrated in fundus photographs by Schmidt and Trojan and in histologic sections by Sourdille (1964) and Hervouet (1968). These latter called this type of haemorrhage "perles jacobines" (cf. explanation of this unusual expression in the Appendix of this book). Even though histologically these submembranacious haemorrhages were found under the internal limiting membrane, they were called "preretinal". An observation by Drews and Minckler (1933) is unusual in this respect: A haemorrhage of 10 disc diameters under the internal limiting membrane was resorbed after 6 days. A gradual evaluation of retinal haemorrhage caused by subarachnoid haemorrhage is given by Fahmy (1972a), but his morphologic classification, too, cannot be accepted: Streaked haemorrhages in the nerve fibre layer, round haemorrhages on the surface and flame-shaped haemorrhages subretinally.

Frequently these haemorrhages invade the vitreous body (Riddoch and Goulden, 1925; Drews and Minckler, 1944; Aust et al., 1967; Schmidt and Trojan, 1970; Göttinger, 1971; Duke-Elder, 1971). Vitreous haemorrhage caused by subarachnoid haemorrhage is also called "Terson syndrome" (Terson, 1926; Paunoff, 1962; Castren, 1963; von Grósz, 1966; Khan and Frenkel, 1975). Vessel ruptures have been seen in histologic preparations (Ballantyne, 1943; Miller and Cuttino, 1948).

This postnatal type of retinal haemorrhage is a most important symptom and indicator of intracranial haemorrhage. Dolcet-Buxeres and Ferrer-Pi (1964) reported on a child without retinal haemorrhage after caesarian section. Retinal haemorrhage occurred accompanying the manifestations of an intracranial haemorrhage at the 15th day. Occurrence of intracranial and retinal haemorrhage together was reported in 1/2 (1964) or 2/3 of the cases (1966) by Sourdille. Schmidt and Trojan (1970) found them in 40% of their cases, Fahmy (1973) in 90% of his fatal cases. Sequelae are possible. Fahmy (1972b) reports on macular disorders, which he connects with break down products of haemoglobin and not with a direct macular haemorrhage.

Symonds (1924) believed that vitreous haemorrhages, in cases of intracranial haemorrhage, are caused by a direct penetration of blood through the lamina cribrosa. This opinion (discussed also by Paunoff, 1962) is not supported by histologic investigations by other authors, who found the lamina cribrosa intact (Riddoch and Goulden, 1925; MacDonald, 1931; Greear, 1943; Drews and Minckler, 1944; Miller and

Cuttino, 1948; Göttinger, 1971). Manschot (1951, 1954) experimented with ink injections into the subarachnoid space. He proved that the cerebrospinal fluid spaces are contiguous even when the space at the foramen opticum is very narrow. Adhesions would explain why blood is not regularly found in the sheaths of the optic nerve in subarachnoid haemorrhage. Smith et al. (1957) considered that blood found behind the eye ball need not necessarily have penetrated along the optic nerve sheaths but that the distant effects of intracranial pressure could cause haemorrhage within the sheaths themselves.

It is of primary interest that the elevation of intracranial pressure and its build-up in the dural sheaths of the optic nerve can cause papilloedema as well as retinal haemorrhage. We observed one case in which haemorrhages of the nerve fibre layer had slightly elevated the internal limiting membrane, and haemorrhages of the internal granular layer had invaded the external plexiform layer, even penetrating the external limiting membrane. Experiments in dogs (Cushing and Bordley, 1909; Wolf and Davies, 1931; Smith et al., 1957) have not been successful in producing true papilloedema because of the different vascularization of the canine disc. In the rhesis monkey Smith et al. (1957) produced retinal haemorrhage, including one submembranacious haemorrhage (which they called preretinal). Hayreh (1964) also experimented with the rhesus monkey and produced papilloedema and retinal haemorrhage by raising intracranial pressure. It is of great interest that the disc did not respond in proportion to measured intracranial pressure change. Variations in the degree of patency of the sheath of the optic nerve, especially in the area of the optic canal, seem to influence the conveying of cerebrospinal fluid in the optic nerve sheath.

True papilloedema seems to require some time for its formation, e.g. 10 min (?) according to Niedermeier (1956), or 2 h according to a clinical observation by Zehetbauer (1977). The impairment of axoplasmic transport (Mickler and Tso, 1976), causing swelling of the disc, certainly occurs so slowly that it cannot be caused by perinatal elevation of cerebrospinal fluid pressure within optic nerve sheaths.

The elevation of pressure in the central retinal vein plays the major part in the pathogenesis of retinal haemorrhage or papilloedema due to increased intracranial pressure. Measurements by Hedges et al. (1964) demonstrated that when " . . . the cerebrospinal fluid pressure reached the level of the systemic arterial blood pressure . . . , the veins became engorged and the venous haemorrhages appeared in the posterior pole of the fundus".

Where does obstruction of the central retinal vein take place? The schematic drawing from Miller and Cuttino (1948) in Figure 62 demonstrates how transmitted pressure of the cerebrospinal fluid reaches the vein when it passes from the optic nerve into the dural sheaths through the subarachnoid space. Miller and Cuttino also point to anastomoses of choroidal vessels with the central retinal artery and vein, behind the lamina cribrosa [which according to François and Neetens (1965) are of little importance]. The vein is said to pass through the subarachnoid space more obliquely than the artery. It can be extended by subdural pressure so that its lumen narrows (MacDonald, 1931).

The importance of these points has been exaggerated. The most significant fact is that elevated intracranial pressure is transmitted through the dural sheaths of the optic nerve as far as the lamina cribrosa. The entire content of the dural sheath is

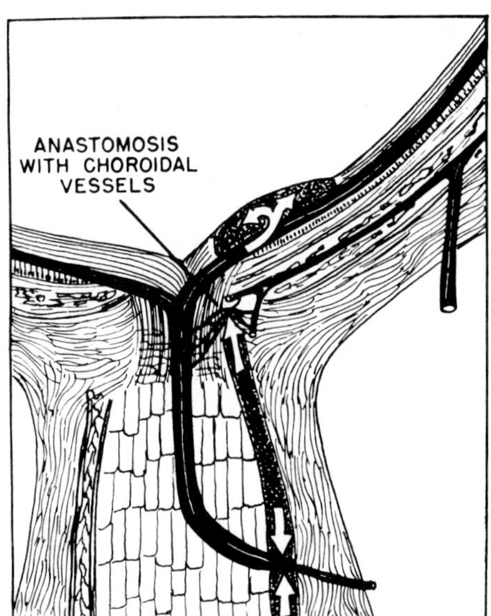

Fig. 62. Schematic drawing from Miller and Cuttino (1948). Elevated pressure of cerebrospinal fluid will compress central retinal vein and choroidal anastomoses behind lamina cribrosa

uniformly exposed to pressure, which obstructs venous outflow more than arterial input. In considering perinatal retinal haemorrhage these haemodynamic factors must be kept in mind.

3. Trauma

Nobiling (1884) found retinal haemorrhage in suffocated newborn infants. It remains unclear whether the haemorrhages were sequelae of strangulation or perinatal in origin. Experimentally Metzger (1925) tried to produce retinal haemorrhage in young dogs and rabbits by suffocation, strangulation and application of negative pressure to the cranium. In most cases he could produce retinal haemorrhage. Liebrecht (1906) found retinal haemorrhage in cases of cranial fracture. Such traumatic haemorrhages seem to have been very little studied in comparison to perinatal ones.

Of special interest are those connected with the battered baby syndrome. In most cases they occur together with intracranial haemorrhage (Aaron et al., 1970; Caffey, 1974; Harcourt and Hopkins, 1973), but Harcourt and Hopkins (1971) also report on children with retinal haemorrhage without subdural effusion. They saw macular and other retinal scars as sequelae. This is of interest because the differences between perinatal haemorrhages and those occurring in the battered syndrome are a question of degree. Further observations of retinal sequelae in this syndrome would be of great help.

4. Summary

Retinal haemorrhage in the newborn must be compared to three other types of retinal haemorrhage. All these originate from increased pressure of the central retinal vein. This, in the first type, is caused by venous occlusion which, in fresh and incomplete stages, produces the same types of haemorrhage as in the newborn. A second type is due to elevation of cerebrospinal fluid pressure as in intracranial haemorrhage. The intracranial pressure transmitted to the dural sheath of the optic nerve obstructs venous outflow, and, when longer lasting, causes papilloedema. But a sequel to acute elevation of intracranial pressure, also in experiments, is typical retinal haemorrhaging. The third type, due to trauma, is partly connected with subarachnoid haemorrhage, but it seems that it can also appear independently. More observations are necessary, especially of retinal scar formation in the battered baby syndrome.

Zusammenfassung

Die Netzhautblutungen beim Neugeborenen müssen mit 3 anderen retinalen Blutungen verglichen werden, die durch erhöhten Druck in der Zentralvene auftreten.

1. Der Zentralvenenverschluß zeigt besonders im frischen oder unvollständigen Stadium die gleichen morphologischen Typen von Blutungen wie beim Neugeborenen.

2. Druckerhöhung des Liquor cerebrospinalis wie bei intracraniellen Blutungen wird entlang den Opticusscheiden fortgeleitet und behindert den venösen Ausfluß. Bei längerem Bestehen tritt eine Stauungspapille auf, bei kurzfristiger Erhöhung des intracraniellen Druckes, auch bei Experimenten, treten typische Neuthautblutungen auf.

3. Durch Trauma, teilweise zu Subarachnoidalblutung führend, jedoch wohl auch unabhängig erscheinend, können vergleichbare Netzhautblutungen auftreten. Weitere Beobachtungen besonders der Narbenbildung in der Netzhaut beim Battered Baby Syndrom wären notwendig.

F. Correlation with Other Perinatal Haemorrhages

During birth, conjunctival and choroidal haemorrhages can occur, which should be compared to perinatal retinal haemorrhages. Another specific type of haemorrhage is the cephalhaematoma; this has also been studied in connection with retinal haemorrhage.

1. Cephalhaematoma

The cephalhaematoma is caused by negative pressure on the parts of the head which have already left the birth canal. A correlation with the frequency of retinal haemorrhage was not found by Stumpf and von Sicherer (1909), Yamanouchi (1959), Ishikawa (1959), Koyama (1959), Bachmann et al. (1968). Mezey (1952) stresses that cephalhaematoma is frequent in immature children, whereas retinal haemorrhage is not. A positive correlation is reported only by Kawakami et al. (1963), but in a very small series.

Thus, formation of a cephalhaematoma seems to be connected with circulatory conditions that are not the same as those causing perinatal retinal haemmorrhage.

2. Conjunctival Haemorrhages

A few authors compare the occurrences of retinal and conjunctival haemorrhage. Table 27 gives the details from four authors. No correlation of the two can be found from this table. This is also confirmed by Aliquò-Mazzei (1966) and Jochmus (1968). A higher number of conjunctival haemorrhages was found by François and Tranos (1975) under microscopic examination, but here also no correlation was seen.

Table 27. Correlation of retinal and conjunctival haemorrhages

Author	Year	Conj. haem. ∅		Conj. haem. +	
		Ret. haem. ∅	Ret. haem. +	Ret. haem. ∅	Ret. haem. +
Koyama	1959	322/510=63%	115/510=23%	45/510= 9%	18/510= 4%
Baum and Bulpitt	1970	150/210=71%	31/210=15%	27/210=13%	2/210= 1%
Wierhake	1971	44%	28%	17%	11%

Baum and Bulpitt (1970) found a positive correlation between conjunctival haemorrhage and birth weight, cranial circumference, gestation period, short second stage of labour, high Apgar score and high parity. They could find no correlation between these criteria and retinal haemorrhage in their series, consisting mainly of immature infants. The uniqueness of the circulatory conditions of the retina is pointed out by the lack of correlation between haemorrhage in two areas so closely related.

3. Choroidal Haemorrhages

Perinatal choroidal haemorrhages seem to be very rare. Naumoff (1890) found three cases. Coburn (1904) saw one choroidal effusion that penetrated Bruch's membrane and lifted the retina. In our histologic material, no such haemorrhage could be found. Even if with transillumination a denser area of the choroid was visible, engorged choroidal vessels were still intact in the sections. We could also find no choroidal effusion on funduscopic examination. A darker choroidal area, temporal and below the macula, frequently seen in the light background of the newborn, corresponds to a long ciliary artery. Ehlers et al. (1974) report on some peripheral choroidal haemorrhages, but without an exact definition.

Iris haemorrhages or hyphaema have been mentioned by Coburn (1904), Kauffman (1941), Brogi et al. (1962) and Ciehanowska (1964).

4. Summary

Perinatal haemorrhages due to elevated blood pressure in the infantile head — cephalhaematoma, conjunctival and choroidal haemorrhages — have not been found to be positively correlated with retinal haemorrhage. This latter depends on special circulatory conditions that cannot be explained only by an elevation of the blood pressure in the head.

Zusammenfassung

Perinatale Blutungen, die durch den erhöhten Blutdruck im Bereich des kindlichen Kopfes erklärt werden, wie Kephalhämatom, conjunctivale und chorioidale Blutungen, sind nicht positiv mit Netzhautblutungen korreliert. Letztere werden durch besondere Kreislaufbedingungen hervorgerufen, die nicht nur in einer Blutdruckerhöhung des Schädels bestehen.

G. Aetiology and Pathogenesis

1. Literature

With the first description of perinatal retinal haemorrhages in 1881, Königstein presented the first hypothesis about their origin. He believed them to be caused by the arteriolization of infantile blood after the first inspiration. This idea was later dismissed.

Schleich (1884) and Berger (1892) beliebed that blockage of circulation during deformation of the foetal head was the cause. In 1890 Naumoff stated in his excellent paper that mere congestion of the foetal head could not be the only cause for retinal haemorrhage. He felt in this case that choroidal and conjunctival haemorrhages would occur with the same frequency. He was the first to consider the pressure of the cerebrospinal fluid to be of importance: With the elevation of intracranial pressure during delivery, the pressure of the cerebrospinal fluid is transmitted through the subarachnoid spaces of the optic nerve and acts upon the central retinal vessels. The retinal circulation differs from that of other surrounding tissues in the passage of these vessels through the sheaths of the optic nerve. Though this idea is certainly valid, it was attacked by von Hippel (1898), who stated that the spaces for cerebrospinal fluid within the optic nerve sheaths were narrow and somtimes even lacking. Several authors followed this line of thought, though it contains an important error. If in a certain number of newborn infants, no passage into the optic nerve sheaths of cerebrospinal fluid were possible, this would be an explanation for the irregular and unpredictable occurrence of perinatal retinal haemorrhage. These latter are not constantly found under predisposing conditions like asphyxia or certain obstetric procedures. In addition Coburn (1904) said that a temporary dilatation of the subdural spaces during delivery might not necessarily be visible in histologic sections. Much later Hayreh (1964) confirmed with his experiments that there are individual differences in the patency of the optic nerve sheaths.

A survey of other early opinions about the origin of perinatal retinal haemorrhages follows:

Paul (1900): Retina subject to haemorrhage because of its delicate tissue and few anastomoses.

Thomson and Buchanan (1903): Increase of blood pressure caused by obstruction of the placentar circulation or sudden relaxation of extreme pressure in the head " . . . allowing the full force of the blood to come suddenly into relaxed vessels may give rise to haemorrhages in the retina and choroid in certain cases."

Berger and Loewy (1906): Toxaemia with disturbance of placentar circulation; elevation of blood pressure with venous congestion.

Seefelder (1907): Compression of the cranium.

Stumpf and von Sicherer (1909): Inhibition of circulation under the special pressure conditions during birth.

Ehrenfest (1922): Anatomic conditions, e.g. the vena centralis retinae emptying anastomoses into the cavernous sinus; fragility of retinal vessels in premature infants; abnormal coagulability of the blood of the newborn.

Although in this monograph it was attempted to collect all important material, it would be impossible to discuss all aetiologic factors proposed by so many authors. Too many investigators have added new aspects to the discussion, mainly trying to explain their own findings.

The author wishes to end the chronologic compilation here and to arrange additional opinions in categories. These will be grouped according to key words, which summarize the aetiologic factors considered to be important by the following authors.

a) Elevation of Intracranial Pressure

The effect of intracranial pressure, which is connected with the effect of birth on retinal circulation, is discussed as the leading factor by: Rico (1939), Kauffman (1941), Giles (1960), Brogi et al. (1962), Sanchez-Ibanez (1963), Jain and Gupta (1965), Moulène (1965), Schenker and Gombos (1966), Neuweiler and Onwudiwe (1967), Sachsenweger (1967), Takeda (1968), Braendstrup (1969), Hoo (1973), François and Tranos (1975).

Other obstetric factors have been dealt with in the chapters on different types of delivery. Still others have been discussed:

Pressure alterations after the ruptur of the foetal membranes: Candian (1949), Konstantopais (1956), Pommer (1972)

Spasm of interior segment of the uterus or pressure of the cervix: Sanchez-Ibanez (1963), Ciehanowsky et al. (1974), Zgorzalewicz (1974)

Decreased pressure after delivery of the head: Metzger (1925)

Compression of jugular veins: Dolcet-Buxeres and Ferrer-Pi (1954), Moulène (1965), Fritz et al. (1966)

Retinal stasis by compression of the thorax: Ehlers et al. (1974)

b) Vascular Factors

Different aspects of the condition of foetal vessels have been discussed:

Endothelial conditions: Falls and Jurow (1946)
Tendency for ruptures, especially in premature infants: Yoshioka (1954)
Disturbances of capillary permeability by stress of birth: Cavrot (1956)
Fragility of capillaries due to a decrease in oestrogen hormones: Gajaria et al. (1965)

c) Anoxia

Asphyxia or anoxia with subsequent vessel dilatation is discussed as being important by Falls and Jurow (1946), Jirman (1947), Millán and Beltrán (1950), Sanchez-Ibañez (1963), Krauer-Mayer (1965b), Takeda (1968), Tranou-Sphalangakou (1968), Evsyukova (1969), Krause et al. (1964) (cf. Tables 25 and 26).

d) Haemorrhagic Diathesis

The differing opinions concerning the haematologic conditions of the newborn have been discussed in Chap. VII, Sect. D.

e) Anatomic Conditions

The special anatomic conditions of retinal circulation and drainage (von Barsewisch, 1975) have been discussed mainly in connection with papilloedema (Chap. VII, Sect. E.2). Only a few authors have discussed the matter in connection with retinal haemorrhage, e.g. Juler (1937) on the connection of the central retinal vein to the cavernous sinus.

A very important aspect, published by Brückner et al. (1949), seems to have been entirely overlooked in the literature: He associates the pressure elevation within the optical nerve sheaths already discussed with the pressure conditions of the internal carotid artery. With elevation of the intracranial pressure, blood will avoid entering the cranium and choose instead the only extracranial branch, i.e. the opthalmic artery.

In the extreme the ophthalmic artery functionally becomes the main and final branch of the internal carotid artery and in its area supplied an arterial plethora will result which can be produced by no other way in equal intensity during spontaneous physio-pathological processes.

This literary survey of the factors considered to cause perinatal retinal haemorrhage, as mentioned before, is incomplete, merely listing ideas and key words that have been discussed, and omitting some of the more exotic theories.

2. Discussion

It is obvious from the foregoing sections that no signle factor can be found to cause or prevent perinatal retinal haemorrhage. A selection from the many ideas has to be made, and the clinical data have to be evaluated not of a single series (in most cases too small), but from many series.

As a basis for discussion, the clinical facts will be repeated in a simplified and concise form:

a)   The retinal haemorrhages discussed occur during labour.
b)   They are caused by rhexis of retinal venules and capillaries.
c)   The greatest similarity can be found to other haemorrhages resulting from venous outflow obstruction, i.e. central venous occlusion or venous obstruction in intracranial pressure elevation by pressure transmitted within the sheaths of the optic nerve.
d)   No correlation exists with other perinatal ocular haemorrhages, like choroidal or conjunctival effusions.
e)   Altering the coagulability of foetal blood seems to be of no influence on the incidence; drugs supporting capillary resistance may be of influence.
f)   With spontaneous delivery from occipital presentation about 1/3 of newborns have retinal haemorrhages.
g)   If the cranium is compressed after the body is released (breech presentation), haemorrhages are rare; if the cranium is not compressed (caesarian section) they are also rare but seem to occur with asphyxia or attempted labour.
h)   Use of vacuum extraction, forceps delivery and pituitary preparations are correlated with a higher incidence of haemorrhage but also with prolonged labour and, frequently, intrauterine asphyxia. Also the influence of parity and age of the mother seem to be based on prolonged second stages of labour.
i)   Asphyxia is a predisposing factor.

As a result of these considerations, the pathogenesis must be based on two principal factors:

a)   Anoxia with vessel dilatation
b)   Compression of the cranium producing pressure elevation within retinal vessels via
     1. Arterial inflow
     2. Pressure of the cerebrospinal fluid
     3. Venous outflow

Compression of the soft foetal cranium causes high intracranial pressure. The internal carotid artery expresses most of its blood into the only extracranial branch, the ophthalmic artery. As regards the arterial blood supply, the retina is exposed to the same conditions as the choroid or the conjunctiva. These areas, also, suffer from a certain obstruction of venous drainage but anastomosize to surrounding venous systems. Contrary to this, the central retinal vein drains into the cavernous sinus, which itself is exposed to the highly elevated intracranial pressure. In addtion to this, the elevated pressure of the cerebrospinal fluid is transmitted to the sheaths of the optic nerve. Within the dural space, the contents, especially the central retinal vein inside and outside the optic nerve, are compressed. This cannot be prevented by the insignificant anastomoses with choroidal veins. The result is engorgement and ruptures in the venous system, and extravasation until pressure conditions change and fibrinous thrombi occlude the ruptures. No papilloedema can form within the short time in which retinal haemorrhage occurs, though the basic conditions have many details in common. Since vessels are more subject to rupture if dilated by anoxia, it is evident that even less traumatic courses of delivery may lead to retinal haemorrhage. On the other hand, without anoxia, prevailing elevated pressure conditions may also lead to haemorrhage.

These mechanisms are not always adequate to explain why a haemorrhage does or does not appear. An important third factor is individual anatomic variations, such as

1. Differences of patency of subdural spaces in optic nerve sheaths
2. Variants of choroidal anastomoses of the central retinal vein
3. Variants of the course of the central retinal vein towards the cavernous sinus
4. Individual differences in vascular fragility, possibly depending on stage of maturity

These factors are difficult to study. Other items of minor importance might also influence or modify retinal haemorrhage: Only after delivery of the head could thoracic compression or compression of the jugular veins elevate cranial blood pressure. This may cause conjunctival haemorrhage and, possibly, further bleeding from retinal vessel ruptures. Insufficient coagulability might cause larger haemorrhages by preventing early formation of fibrin thrombi.

Zusammenfassung

a) Die Blutungen treten während der Geburt auf.
b) Sie werden durch Rhexis retinaler Venolen und Kapillaren hervorgerufen.
c) Sie sind am meisten vergleichbar mit anderen Blutungen, die durch Stauung der Zentralvene entstehen.
d) Mit anderen perinatalen Augenblutungen wie chorioidalen oder conjunctivalen Blutungen besteht keine Korrelation.
e) Veränderung der Koagulabilität des kindlichen Blutes scheint ohne Einfluß auf die Frequenz zu sein, Medikamente zur Erhöhung der Kapillarresistenz sind vielleicht von Einfluß.
f) Bei Spontangeburt aus Hinterhauptslage haben etwa 1/3 der Neugeborenen Netzhautblutungen.
g) Wenn der Schädel erst nach Entlastung des Körpers (Beckenendlage) komprimiert wird, sind Blutungen selten; wird der Schädel nicht komprimiert (Kaiserschnitt), sind sie selten und scheinen mit Asphyxie und Geburtsversuch korreliert zu sein.
h) Vakuum-Extraktion, Zangenentbindung und Hypophysenpräparate sind mit erhöhter Blutungsfrequenz, jedoch auch mit erhöhter Geburtsdauer und häufig intrauteriner Asphyxie korreliert. Auch der Einfluß der Parität und des Alters der Mutter scheint über die verlängerte Austreibungperiode einzuwirken.
i) Asphyxie ist ein prädisponierender Faktor.

Die Pathogenese basiert auf 2 prinzipiellen Faktoren:

a) Anoxie mit Gefäßerweiterung
b) Schädelkompression ruft Blutdrucksteigerung in den Netzhautgefäßen hervor über
    1. den arteriellen Zustrom
    2. Liquordruckerhöhung
    3. den venösen Abfluß.

Die Kompression des weichen kindlichen Kopfes ruft eine intracranielle Drucksteigerung hervor. Darauf wird die A. carotis interna ihr Blut hauptsächlich dem ein-
zigen extracraniellen Ast, der A. ophthalmica zuführen. Bezüglich des arteriellen Zu-
stromes wären Retina, Chorioidea und Conjunctiva noch den gleichen Bedingungen
ausgesetzt. Auch diese letzteren werden eine intravasale Drucksteigerung erleben, ihr
Venensystem anastomosiert jedoch mit anderen Systemen der Umgebung. Im Gegensatz dazu fließt die V. centralis retinae ausschließlich in den Sinus cavernosus, der
bereits dem erhöhten intracraniellen Druck ausgesetzt ist. Zusätzlich wird der erhöhte
Liquordruck in den Opticusscheiden weitergeleitet und damit ihr Inhalt, insbesondere
die Zentralvene innerhalb und außerhalb des Sehnerven komprimiert. Dieses können
die unbedeutenden Anastomosen mit Chorioidalgefäßen nicht verhindern. Das Ergeb-
nis sind Erweiterung und schließlich Rupturen des venösen Systems, Extravasationen,
bis die Druckbedingungen sich ändern und Fibrinpfröpfe die Rupturen verschließen.

VIII. Significance

A. Evaluation of Different Types of Delivery

Here it should be repeated that, e.g. in the case of vacuum extraction, the correlation of this procedure with a high incidence of retinal haemorrhage does not indicate that this procedure should be considered hazardous. Always the indication for intervention has to be taken into consideration.

A low Apgar score is correlated with retinal haemorrhages and these may therefore serve as one of several symptoms to establish the diagnosis "asphyxia". But without further studies, it seems too early to evaluate, for instance, electronic monitoring of delivery by estimating the degree of asphyxia from retinal haemorrhages, as Krause et al. (1974) have done.

The details of the correlation of retinal haemorrhage with different types of delivery have been given in Chap. VII.

B. Retinal and Intracranial Haemorrhages

1. Pathoanatomy

Jacobs was the first to assume in the year 1928 that intracranial haemorrhage, so important in the mortality of newborns, might be correlated with perinatal retinal haemorrhage. He examined 14 infants, stillborn or having died a few days after birth, and he found retinal haemorrhages in 12 of these. One immature and 5 mature infants, without intracranial lesions, had only a few retinal haemorrhages; 6 infants with intracranial lesions all had quite severe retinal haemorrhages.

The idea of the positive correlation of retinal with intracranial haemorrhage was studied by several authors: Cavrot (1955, 1956) found the clinical signs of intracranial haemorrhage only in children who had retinal haemorrhages at the same time. He considered the retina to be a model of cerebral processes, depending on the same vascularization and exposed to the same conditions that cause cerebral haemorrhage. Because of the connection of retinal circulation and intracerebral vessels, other authors also postulated a positive correlation: Edgerton (1934), Drozdowa (1951, Sorsby (1963), Kobayashi et al. (1964), Murillo and Murillo (1968), Vincenti and Gavinelli (1969). Bahn (1926) compared the retinal vessels to those of the ventricles.

The authors who have published observations are grouped in Table 28. Some of the diagnoses were established only by clinical methods. Not all papers report in detail on the children with a negative correlation for the two types of bleeding. But this negative correlation is more frequently found than would be expected from Jacobs' report.

Table 28. Intracranial lesion and retinal haemorrhages

Author	Year	Intracranial lesion +		Intracranial lesion ∅	
		Retinal haemorrhages +	Retinal haemorrh. ∅	Retinal haemorrh. +	Retinal haemorrh. ∅
Jacobs	1928	3740 g, intracranial haemorrhage, laceration of falx and left tentorium; engorgement in choroid, retinal haemorrhages		2880 g, few retinal haemorrhages	1950 g, macerated foetus
		2720 g, tear of falx and tentorium; no intracranial haemorrhages. Few retinal haemorrhages		5 mature infants with few retinal	2110 g, spina bifida and meningocele
		2270 g, tear near centre of falx, laceration of tentorium; some retinal haemorrhages			
		3 forceps deliveries: 3330 g, laceration of tentorium, retinal haemorrhages			
		2590 g, laceration of falx, extensive retinal haemorrhages			
		2460 g, intracranial haemorrhage, laceration of tentorium; large retinal haemorrhages			
Eades	1929	3 infants dying within 3 days of intracranial haemorrhage; massive retinal haemorrhages		1 stillborn, cord around neck, retinal and vitreous haemorrhage	
		1 clinical symptom of intracranial pressure			
Sykes	1931	3 dying from intracranial haemorrhage; 2 with light, 1 with massive retinal haemorrhages	2 dying from intra-cranial haemor-rhage		

Kauffman	1941	2 dying from intracranial haemorrhage 2 clinical diagnoses of intracranial haemorrhage	3 clinical diagnoses 3 haemorrhages in cerebrospinal fluid		
Millán and Beltrán	1950		1 mature, 1 immature dying from intra-cranial haemorrhage		
Canon	1952	2 with microscopic haemorrhages in mesencephalon 1 immature, ventricular haemorrhage			1 case
Dolcet	1954	1 case	1 case		
Yoshioka	1954	2 cases	3 cases	8 cases	1 case
Štefek	1956	1 mature child with intracranial haemorrhage	3 mature, 6 immature children		9 mature, 7 immature children
Koyama	1959	1 immature, 2 mature children after forceps delivery		2 cases	2 cases
Motohashi	1960	2 cases with massive retinal haemorrhages			
Brogi et al.	1962	2 with clinical diagnosis			
Blanc	1967	1 clinical diagnosis, 1 dying from intra-cranial haemorrhage; both with massive retinal haemorrhages			
Braendstrup	1969	4 severe and 2 light cerebral lesions with massive retinal haemorrhages. 6 medium and 8 light cerebral lesions with light retinal haemorrhages	5 severe and 22 light cerebral lesions	3 severe, 3 light retinal haemorrhages	

Keeping in mind how unreliable such a method is, we can still add up the values of this table. We find intracranial lesions occurring in 53 cases with retinal haemorrhage and in 50 cases without, absence of intracranial lesions in 23 cases with retinal haemorrhage and in 22 cases without. A correlation seems very unlikely. The material published cannot usefully be compared. Braendstrup (1969) does not clearly separate clinical and autoptic diagnoses. Štefek (1956) reports on a series of mainly immature infants. Doege (1969) found no correlation between intracranial and retinal haemorrhage. The material of Szirmák et al. (1971) shows no tendencies at all.

2. Clinical Examinations

Tanaka (1968) found lateral differences in the electroencephalogram of children with and without retinal haemorrhage. Larsen (1969) found a relative correspondence between retinal haemorrhage, neurologic aberration, and EEG alteration. No reliable correlation has been found by Bachmann et al. (1968), Hickl et al. (1969) and Orduña and de Arizcun (1970). A short note by Figueroa (1958), reporting on 77% retinal haemorrhage with cerebral lesions, is lacking all detail. Cranial fissures or fractures after vacuum extraction seem also to demonstrate no clear correlation with retinal haemorrhage (Bachmann et al., 1968).

3. Discussion

The poor correlation of retinal with intracranial haemorrhage is not surprising if one considers their pathogenesis. The circulatory conditions of the retina during delivery cannot be compared with those of the brain. The venous outflow is exposed to conditions that exist in no other vascularized area of the infant's body. In addition, a further differentiation of intracranial haemorrhage is of importance. With mature infants, lacerations of the tentorium, due to birth trauma, play the major role. In immature infants, subarachnoid, leptomeningeal, para- and intraventricular haemorrhages are of importance (Capper, 1928; Schwartz, 1961; Joppich and Schulte, 1968). According to these authors, 30% of newborn infants dying in West Germany have pathologic cerebral alterations. Of these alterations, however, only 20% are due to birth trauma, whereas 50%–80% are caused by hypoxia.

The prevalence of non-traumatic, hypoxic haemorrhage in the material of the I. Universitäts-Frauenklinik, Munich, is confirmed by Müschenhorn (1970). In 90% of the immature infants with a birth weight under 2500 g, immature vessels can be expected (Hickl, 1972). The non-traumatic nature of these haemorrhages is also explained by the fact that the small head of the immature infant is less exposed to birth trauma. Lacerations of tentorium and falx and subdural effusions are due to compression of the cranium of mature infants. Their time of onset is the same as that of retinal haemorrhage. The non-traumatic and postnatal haemorrhages of the immature are caused by the vicious circle of hypoxia, cerebral oedema and respiratory distress. They are due to diapedesis. Their postnatal origin was tested by Dyer et al. (1971) with erythrocytes marked with Cr.

Reviewing Table 28 again, with this knowledge, we see that many details are missing. Jacobs (1928) observed three forceps deliveries and two mature infants with intracranial lesions due to birth trauma. The lesions were correlated with retinal haemorrhage. But forceps deliveries alone are often accompanied by retinal haemorrhage. Eades (1929) observed two cases of retinal haemorrhage, where symptoms of intracranial pressure were already present. It cannot be proven whether these retinal haemorrhages were perinatal or connected with intracranial pressure. Nor can this possibility be excluded with other authors.

4. Summary

In contradiction to the idea of several authors, haemodynamic conditions of the retina during delivery are not comparable to those of the brain. Perinatal haemorrhages, therefore, do not serve as an indicator for intracranial bleeding. No correlation could be found with intracranial lesions due to birth trauma or to alterations in the electro-encephalogram.

Non-traumatic cerebral haemorrhage, so often fatal to the immature, is caused by postnatal hypoxia and is due to diapedesis. No correlation here with retinal haemorrhage has been confirmed.

Zusammenfassung

Im Gegensatz zu der Ansicht einiger Autoren sind die hämodynamischen Bedingungen der Netzhaut unter der Geburt nicht mit denen des Gehirns vergleichbar. Netzhautblutungen können deshalb nicht als Indikator für intracranielle Blutungen herangezogen werden. Es konnten auch keine Korrelationen zu geburtstraumatischen intracraniellen Läsionen oder elektroencephalographischen Veränderungen gefunden werden. Die nicht-traumatischen cerebralen Blutungen, oft Todesursache bei Frühgeborenen, werden durch postnatale Hypoxie ausgelöst und sind Diapedeseblutungen. Eine Verbindung zu den perinatalen und durch Rhexis hervorgerufenen Netzhautblutungen wurde nicht bestätigt.

C. Retinal Haemorrhage and Amblyopia

About 2% of the population suffer from amblyopia: reduced visual acuity without visible retinal alterations. In many of these cases a refractive error is the cause, and this condition can ofteh be treated. According to Oliver and Nawratzki (1971), who found 2% amblyopic children among 5329 cases, 1/3 of these remained resistent to therapy. This remaining type of amblyopia, not explained by refractive error and not influenced by treatment, has been related to perinatal retinal haemorrhage.

1. Pathoanatomy

Schleich (1884) considered smaller retinal haemorrhages to be innocuous, whereas larger ones could cause amblyopia by lesion of the retinal structure. Naumoff (1890) was convinced that amblyopia could be caused by retinal haemorrhages: Those of the internal granular layer would cause rupture of nerve fibres, ruptured capillaries would remain occluded, and the developing retina would be very vulnerable. But he very clearly states that macular haemorrhage alone can be of importance later. Von Hippel (1898) found a macular haemorrhage penetrating the external limiting membrane and forming a subretinal effusion. He was sure that this macula would have been functionally damaged afterwards. Coburn (1904) believed that, besides producing disturbances of central fixation, nerve fibre haemorrhages would also damage the retina through ascending and descending degeneration. Commenting on Enoch's lecture on receptor amblyopia, Burian (1959) discussed perinatal haemorrhages of the posterior pole that " . . . might produce a disarrangement in the orientation of the sensory retinal element . . . ".

Many authors have discussed macular haemorrhage as a cause of definite damage: Truc (1898), Thomson and Buchanan (1903), Fuchs (1905), Lagrange and Valude (1906), Ehrenfest (1922), Sykes (1931), Kramer (1931, in the *Handbuch* of Schieck and Brückner), Wille (1946), Cook and Glasscock (1951), Arruga (1955), Sorsby (1963), Aliquo-Mazzei (1966), von Noorden and Maumenee (1971).

Paul, in 1900, saw that not every case of amblyopia can be related to birth trauma. He also thought that amblyopia could follow macular haemorrhage. But the improvement of visual acuity by separate training proved that amblyopia could not be exclusively of traumatic origin.

2. Clinical Investigations

a) Original Observations

From the author's material only children with foveolar involvement and with involvement of the macular area were reexamined. At the age of 6 and 7 years, 31 out of 51 children with macular involvement were reexamined (Dissertation: A. Pöllmann, 1979, under the author's supervision). The results concerning visual acuity, binocular function, fixation and funduscopy are given in Table 29. The fundi in all these children have been photographed. Notes and sketches of postnatal examination and, in some cases, postnatal photographs were compared to the current state. For instance, the two submembranacious haemorrhages invading the fovea centralis shown in Figures 39 and 40 should be compared to the later fundus photographs (Figs. 63 and 64). In both cases, not a single trace of irregularity can be found either at the source of bleeding for the flat haemorrhages or at the vessels involved. The outline of the haemorrhagic detachment of the internal limiting membrane is not marked by visible sequelae. Further examples are presented in Plates IV, VI, VIII.

Table 29. Functional results 6 and 7 years after macular haemorrhages

Localisation of haemorrh.	Visual acuity			Titmus test Rings No.			Fixation			Fundus alterations	
	< 0.6	0.7−0.9	1.0	< 3	4−7	8−9	Central	Para-central	?	+	0
Fovea	1	2	15	1	5	10	16	1	1	1	17
Macular border	0	8	22	1	2	12	28	1	1	1	29
Peripheral [a]	0	1	8				8	0	1	1	8
No haemor-rhage [a]	0	0	5				4	0	1	0	5
	62 eyes			31 cases			62 eyes			62 eyes	

a Fellow eyes of cases with macular involvement.

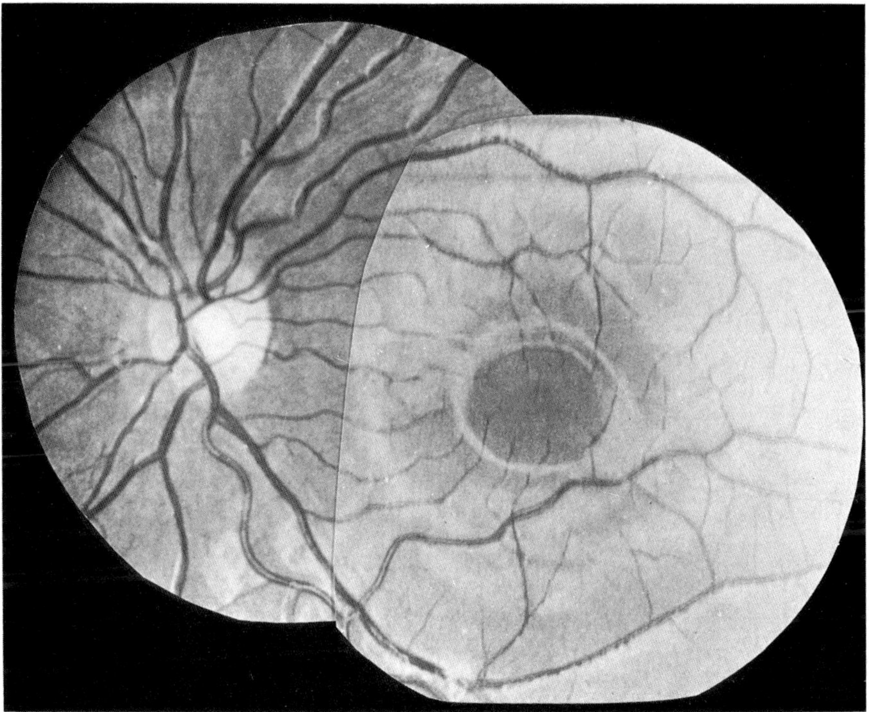

Fig. 63. Reexamination of macular haemorrhage at age 6 years (cf. Fig. 39 and Plate V). Vessels somewhat more tortuous than after birth, macula without any irregularities, no particular alterations at sites of earlier haemorrhages

Among the 62 eyes reexamined, there were 3 with fundus alterations that will be analyzed in detail:

1. Right eye: 15 haemorrhages, 1 submembranacious haemorrhage at the inferior temporal border of the macula. At 7 years of age, minimal pigmentary alteration of the fovea (within normal limits, no previous central haemorrhage).

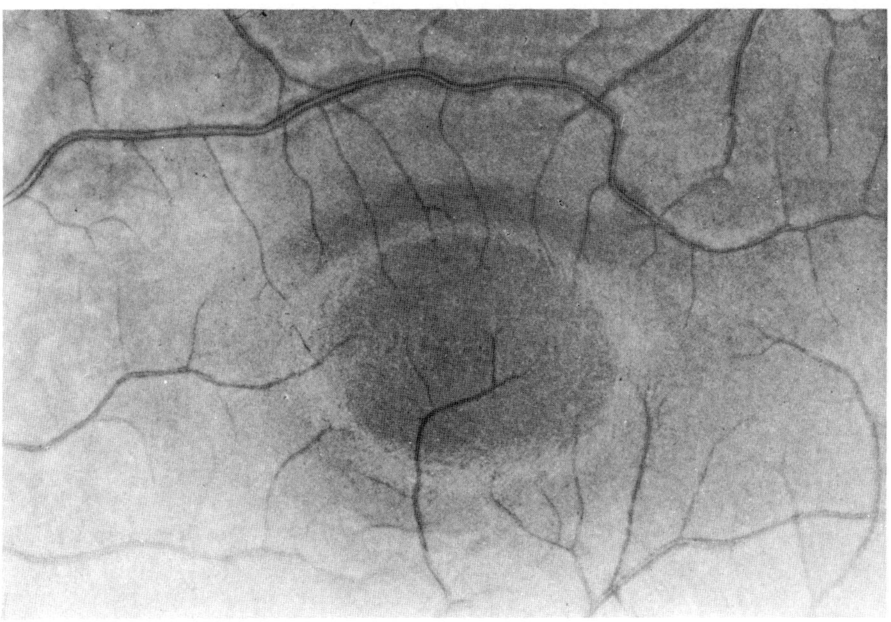

Fig. 64. Reexamination of macular haemorrhage at age 7 years (cf. Plate IX and Fig. 40). Detail photograph of macular area. No irregularities can be seen at site of former haemorrhages

Left eye: 10 haemorrhages, 1 touching the macula from the temporal border. At 7 years of age irregular superficial reflection of the fovea, not coinciding with the original haemorrhage and most probably due to ocular contusion. Visual acuity right eye 0.9, left eye 0.8; Titmus test: Rings Nos. 1–7; fixation: central in both eyes.

2. Right eye (cf. Plate VIII): Massive extensive haemorrhages, one larger submembranacious haemorrhage temporal to the macula. At 6 years of age minimal alteration of superficial retinal reflex at the nasal side of the macula. A choroidal depigmentation is seen in the mid-periphery at 12 o'clock, a region which had not been photographed after birth. A particular type of haemorrhage, e.g. penetration of the external limiting membrane, may have occurred in this area.
Left eye (cf. Plate IX; Figs. 40 and 64): Massive haemorrhages and one very large submembranacious haemorrhage covering the macula. At 6 years of age no irregularities visible. Visual acuity both eyes 1.0: Titmus test: Rings Nos. 1–9; fixation: central in both eyes.

3. Right eye (cf. Plate VI): Massive haemorrhages, one of five submembranacious haemorrhages reaching the fovea from the temporal inferior border. At 7 years of age macula without irregularities.
Left eye (no postnatal photograph): Massive haemorrhages, as on the other side, one submembranacious haemorrhage reaching the fovea from 12 o'clock. At

7 years of age minimal alteration of surface reflection at nasal macular border and minimal pigmentary alteration at inferior border of macula, both without connection to earlier haemorrhages.

Visual acuity both eyes 1.0; Titmus test: Rings Nos. 1–9; fixation: central in both eyes.

4. Another case is of interest. Massive haemorrhage with macular involvement in both eyes. At 6 years of age untreated convergent strabism due to hyperopia of + 2 D in both eyes. Visual acuity improved in the right eye within 3 months of training from 0.4 to 0.6; fixation improved.

In the entire series, foveal involvement was not found to be correlated with visual acuity, binocular function, irregular fixation or ophthalmoscopic alteration. The only case of definite amblyopia was the result of hyperopia and was responsive to treatment. This case had severe haemorrhages, more than 50 extravasations in each eye. The fovea of the right eye was reached by a haemorrhage from the temporal side and, prior to pleoptic treatment at the age of 6 years, fixation centred on the nasal superior border of the fovea. The other eye had a foveal haemorrhage, too, and at the age of 6 years fixation was unsteady but still central. Ophthalmoscopically both maculae were normal. This case does not prove that there is any relationship between the site of foveal haemorrhage and the area of fixation because fixation changed rapidly with treatment.

b) Literature

The first important clinical observation was published by Sidler-Huguenin (1903). In a case of forceps delivery he observed a macular haemorrhage which had persisted for 4 weeks. He reexamined the child at the age of 4.5 years with a good visual acuity and no abnormalities of the macula. Unfortunately, only a few cases report such precise details. A review of the literature is given in Table 30.

The author agrees with the criticism of von Noorden and Khodadoust (1973) that in many cases it is unclear whether cases with macular involvement were reexamined or just cases with retinal haemorrhage. Even when macular involvement was discussed it was sometimes only the macular area and not the fovea that was involved. In the largest series of Pajor et al. (1964) it is uncertain whether cases with macular haemorrhage have a visual function differing from that in cases of peripheral haemorrhage. These authors compared their group of retinal haemorrhages to a normal group with respect to visual acuity and binocular function. But this control group was older than the one with retinal haemorrhage. Besides that, the macular changes found in 11% (fine granulation, loss of superficial reflection) have not been related to macular haemorrhage.

Bonamour (1949) found a random distribution of macular involvement and visual acuity. Two children without macular haemorrhage had decreased visual acuity, and out of 17 children with light and peripheral haemorrhage, one affected eye was amblyopic, certainly unrelated to haemorrhaging. Earlier, irregularities in the macula surface reflex had been observed over a period of months after central haemorrhages (Péhu and Bonamour, 1938).

Table 30. Ophthalmologic follow-up after retinal haemorrhages

Author	Year	Age at reexamination	Cases	Result of ophthalmologic examination	
				at birth	at reexamination
Sidler-Huguenin	1903	4.5 yr	1	Macular haemorrhage after forceps delivery, visible for 4 weeks	v.a [a] good, fundus normal
Jacobs	1928	3.5–5.5 yr	12	Retinal haemorrhages including macular border	v.a. good
			1	Largest haemorrhages fairly close to region of macula	Considerable amblyopia
Jacobs	1930	3.5–5.5 yr	3	Retinal haemorrhages, resorbed within 20 days	1 amblyopia, explained by refractive error
Rowland	1935	2–7 yr	6	Retinal haemorrhages without macular involvement	Fundus normal; examinable with 5: v.a., Haitz, stereoscopic vision or fusion normal
Juler	1937	1–3 yr	5	Macular haemorrhages	Fundus normal, no amblyopia or strabism
Bonamour	1939	1 yr	25	Mainly macular haemorrhages	No macular alterations
Croci and Scardaccione	1941	6–14 mo	14	Macular haemorrhages	Fundus normal; 3 convergent strabism by refractive error
Bonamour	1949	10 yr	8	Macular haemorrhages	7: v.a. good; 1: myopic, v.a. 2/10;
			11	Extended haemorrhages without macular involvement	9: v.a. good; 1: v.a. 5/10; 1: v.a. 2/10
			17	Discrete haemorrhages	14: normal; 1: strabism of involved eye; 2: strabism of fellow eye
Drozdowa	1951	8.5–32 mo	14	Bilateral haemorrhages, 11 with macular involvement	Fundus normal
			1	Macular haemorrhage	Pigment alteration corresponding to the haemorrhage
Konstantopais	1956	8–9 yr	20	Some with macular haemorrhages	Fundus normal, no amblyopia
Duesberg and Tiburtius	1958	ca. 2 yr	15	Retinal haemorrhages	Normal
			1	Bilateral extended haemorrhage	Convergent strabism with hyperopia
			1	Unilateral haemorrhage	Bilateral pigment alterations

Author	Year	Age	n	Finding	Outcome
Mao	1959	4–5 yr	23	Retinal haemorrhages	Fundus normal, v.a. good
Pajor et al.	1964	3 yr	227	Retinal haemorrhages	11% fine granulation of the macula and decreased surface reflex; v.a. examinable in 80% only
Fritz et al.	1966	?	20	Retinal haemorrhages	1 strabism (refraction?)
			1	Macular haemorrhage	Degenerative area of the macula
Krebs and Jäger	1966	1 yr	60	Retinal haemorrhages	Fundus normal, no strabism
Birich and Peretiskaya	1968	3.5–4.5 yr	118	Retinal haemorrhages	Amblyopia and strabism only with refractive error
				Macular involvement	Without influence
Hager	1968	1–2 yr	?	Retinal haemorrhages after vacuum extraction	1 macular pigment alteration
Braendstrup	1969	?	?	Foveal haemorrhage with pigmentation after 2–4 months	Later normal fundus
Remky	1969	4–5 yr	2	Macular haemorrhages	No amblyopia
Richter	1969	11–26 mo	452	With and without haemorrhages	1.6% concomitant strabism; 4.3% periodic or suspected strabism
			?	Macular haemorrhages	No correlation to strabism
Sasaki	1971	6 yr	24	Large haemorrhages, no macular involvement	No amblyopia
			11	Macular haemorrhages	No amblyopia
Lukaszewicz	1972	2–3 yr	14	Macula and macular area	4 with unilateral amblyopia, 5 with retinal scars (where?)
			16	Peripheral haemorrhages	1 with retinal scars (where?)
Gottstein and Schnecke	1973	3–4 yr	211	(Of 416 children with 27.4% retinal haemorrhages)	3.3% manifest, 2.3% latent strabism unconnected with retinal haemorrhages
von Noorden and Khodadoust	1973	4–5 yr	5	Macular haemorrhages	Fundus normal; 4: v.a. good; 1: v.a. 20/30 o.u.

Table 30 (continued)

Author	Year	Age at reexamination	Cases	Result of ophthalmologic examination	
				at birth	at reexamination
Chang	1974	3–6 yr	73	Eyes without haemorrhages, control group	Mean v.a. 0.90
			25	Eyes with retinal haemorrhages, no macular involvement	Mean v.a. 0.94
			18	Eyes with macular haemorrhages	Mean v.a. 0.92
Schenk and Stangler-Zuschrott	1974	3–7 yr	22	After numerous retinal haemorrhages	Macula normal with all cases
				4 years old, bilateral macular haemorrhages after vacuum extraction	v.a. o.d. 3/8, o.s. 3/8, instable fixation
				3.5 years, macular haemorrhage o.s. after cord around the neck	v.a. o.d. 3/6, o.s. 3/12
				5.5 years, macular haemorrhage o.s.	v.a. o.d. 6/6, o.s. 6/12, improving to 6/8, microstrabism o.s.
Lowes et al.	1976	4.5–6.5 yr	38		All fundi normal
				1 bilateral haemorrhage	v.a. o.d. 1.0; o.s. 0.7, convergent strabism with suppression scotoma
				1 macular haemorrhage o.d.	v.a. o.d. 0.7; o.s. 0.9, suppression scotoma o.d.
				1 macular haemorrhage o.s.	v.a. o.d. 1.0; o.s. 0.8
Pöllmann	1979	6–7 yr	18	Eyes with foveal haemorrhage	1: minimal pigment alterations of both maculae after unilateral macular haemorrhage
					1: changes in surface reflection at the border of the macula, where no previous haemorrhage
					1: amblyopia with hyperopia
			30	Eyes with haemorrhages at the macular border	1: alteration of the surface reflex at the macular border where no previous haemorrhage but contusion

a   v.a., visual acuity.

Comparable to our findings in one case, Duesberg and Tiburtius (1958) report on a case of bilateral pigment alteration of the macula, after unilateral central haemorrhage. With their late examination date (up to the 7th day) it is conceivable that a macular haemorrhage had already been reabsorbed in the other eye.

Of all the observations, there are only three cases with visible macular alterations that have been related to haemorrhage. These are early observations only and lack many details:

Drozdowa (1951): Reexamination of binocular haemorrhages at the age of 8–32 months, one pigment concentration that corresponded to an earlier macular haemorrhage

Fritz et al. (1966); "Sub-macular" haemorrhage resulting in a "degenerative" area several months later

Hager (1968): Macular pigment alterations 1 or 2 years after vacuum extraction (with macular haemorrhage?)

Sachsenweger (1965, 1967) emphasizes that, even without visible sequelae, macular haemorrhages are reabsorbed slowly, often within 1 or 2 months. This could cause an inhibition in the development of the fixation reflex. Even minute haemorrhages may not be harmless in this respect. In addition, the messiness (*"Unsauberkeit"*) of maculae in amblyopic eyes could be connected with earlier haemorrhages. But in 1968 he added: "The statistical relationship between haemorrhages and amblyopia is so vague that one cannot speak of a significant coincidence of the two conditions." Doege (1969) discusses subretinal haemorrhage causing a disturbance of retinal nutrition, intraretinal haemorrhage causing laceration and atrophy of nerve elements and vessel rupture causing vessel occlusion, all based on histologic examination. This last mechanism appears to be of little importance, since the author's examinations demonstrate fibrin thrombi that occlude the vessel rupture but not the lumen of the dilated vessel itself.

Only Vancea (1967) states that amblyopia is a sequel to haemorrhage, without any further details. Kauffman (1958) could find no relation in occasional reexamination of the large series of children he had seen after birth. Franceschetti (1968) found a low incidence of squint in reexaminations. The data of Chang (1974) were given in terms of average visual acuity between ages 3 and 6 years. The average visual acuity was found to be 0.92 in 18 eyes with macular haemorrhage; 0.94 in 25 eyes after retinal haemorrhage in other locations; 0.90 in 73 eyes without haemorrhage. His conclusion is: Macular haemorrhage at birth is not a cause of amblyopia.

One aspect not hitherto discussed was added by Schenk and Stangler-Zuschrott (1974): Four children with reduced fusional amplitude had suffered from extensive thrombosis-like haemorrhages of the posterior pole. The authors discuss a possible connection, since quality of fusion depends on quality of perception in the perimacular retina.

Other reports try to correlate obstetric complications with visual acuity, without observation of perinatal retinal haemorrhages. It must be kept in mind that macular haemorrhages occur in 4% of normal deliveries and in about 25% after vacuum extraction. The incidence is far higher than that of amblyopia in the population. Unger found obstetric complications in 45% of 300 children with strabism. Sachsenweger (1965) estimates the percentage of severe forms or amblyopia, not accessible to early treatment, to be 10%–20%. His attempt to correlate success of early treatment with complications of gestation and birth was without clear result.

Other sequelae have been discussed: Edgerton (1934) thought that macular changes can cause amblyopia, congenital nystagmus and degenerative macular alterations. Velhagen (1964) connects peripheral haemorrhages with pigmentary alterations of otherwise unclear genesis. Coloboma has been discussed by Coburn (1904), retinoblastoma by Wehrli (1905), Coat's disease by Vancea (1941). A few observations of severe hayaloid haemorrhage, mainly in premature infants, make it likely that important sequelae persist (Braendstrup, 1969).

3. Discussion

Perinatal macular haemorrhage as a possible cause of amblyopia should be discussed with respect to the histologic details published in this monograph. Vessel ruptures and subsequent occlusions by fibrin thrombi could cause temporary disturbances in minute areas of retinal circulation. No fluorescein angiographs have been carried out in newborn infants, so that the importance of vessel obstruction is not known clinically. Histologic examinations have not yet proven that tissue damage actually occurs. The sections presented in this work suggest that fibrin thrombi do not cause a complete obliteration of venules; capillary occlusions, however, might be possible.

With a vessel rupture in the nerve fibre layer and the ganglion cell layer, three changes in the tissue occur:

1.   Extension of virtual spaces along the nerve fibres
2.   Extension of virtual perivascular spaces
3.   Detachment of the internal limiting membrane in submembranacious haemorrhages

With a capillary rupture in the internal nuclear layer there are also three possible changes:

1.   Dislocation of cells of the internal nuclear layer
2.   Rupture of the internal plexiform layer, rarely seen
3.   Penetration into the external granular layer or possible rupture of the external limiting membrane

All these developments of retinal haemorrhage cannot originate in the avascular macula itself – a fact that has hardly been discussed in the literature. Every haemorrhage covering the fovea has as its source a perimacular haemorrhage. The most frequent or possibly the only type of haemorrhage reaching the fovea is the submembranacious type, as a result of limited space in the nerve fibre layer. Possibly, the structure of the Müller cells permits easier detachment of the internal limiting membrane of the foveal retina; we must ask ourselves whether this lesion is important. The histologic findings after reattachment of the internal limiting membrane are unknown. Since in the macular area deeper layers are hardly involved, discussion of a malorientation of sensory elements is hypothetical.

Even if visible sequelae of macular haemorrhage are extremely rare, a central haemorrhage totally inhibits the macula for weeks and sometimes for months. Here functional damage is only a question of length of time of resorption. Clinical reports do not contain enough details to clarify this possibility in some cases.

Haemorrhages that cause destruction of nerve tissue, without the possibility of regeneration, has to be discussed separately. The separation itself of cells of the internal granular layer could cause lacerations, and a rupture of the internal plexiform layer is bound to result in permanent damage. Ruptures of the external limiting membrane, perhaps rare in surviving children, could disturb the connections between cones and rods and pigment epithelium. But these true subretinal haemorrhages, observed in histologic sections, cannot be found in clinical descriptions, probably because of problems of terminology. Such are subretinal haemorrhages could affect the macula, possibly causing visible damage. Other important lesions bound to the vascularized perimacular retina may cause small scotomas, which have not yet been demonstrated.

Many authors believe that the not yet fully differentiated retinal tissue is especially vulnerable during the perinatal period. The opposite viewpoint seems not to have been discussed: Could the not yet differentiated retina have a greater ability to compensate the sequelae of haemorrhages, e.g. the detachment of the internal limiting membrane as one sequela? What is missing is not only the evaluation of follow-ups after macular haemorrhage, but also photographic documentation and detailed data about location of haemorrhages and fixation. Of particular interest would be a follow-up of the material from Tübingen (Wierhake, 1971) with photographs of all fundi. For the time being, it can only be said that a connection of retinal, and especially macular, haemorrhaging to amblyopia is unlikely. Not all intractable cases can be attributed to retinal haemorrhage. Only a very limited number of macular haemorrhages seem to have caused sequelae.

4. Summary

Peripheral retinal haemorrhages have no influence on the subsequent function of the eye. Some types of haemorrhage causing definite tissue damage have to cause small scotomas. Haemorrhages affecting the macula must have invaded this avascular zone from the vascularized perimacular retina. The typical macular affection, the submembranacious haemorrhage, seems to heal without visible of functional alteration. The detachment of the internal limiting membrane is probably not a severe trauma to the not yet fully differentiated retina. Functional damage due to the exclusion of the macula seems to be rare. The macular fixation reflex develops at a time when even these long-standing haemorrhages have been resorbed. Deficiency of fusional amplitude after "thrombosis-like" perimacular haemorrhages may be possible.

Zusammenfassung

Periphere Netzhautblutungen sind für die spätere Funktion des Auges bedeutungslos. Einzelne Blutungsformen mit eindeutiger Gewebeschädigung müssen kleine Skotome hervorrufen. Maculablutungen können in diese avaskuläre Zone nur von der vaskularisierten, perimacularen Retina eindringen. Die typische Form, eine submembranöse Blutung, scheint ohne sichtbare oder funktionelle Folgen auszuheilen. Die Abhebung der Lamina limitans interna ist wahrscheinlich kein schweres Trauma der noch nicht völlig differenzierten Netzhaut. Funktionelle Schädigung durch die zeitweilige Ausschaltung der Macula scheint selten vorzukommen. Der Fixationsreflex entwickelt sich erst, wenn auch länger bestehende, zentrale Blutungen resorbiert sind. Verringerung der Fusionsbreite nach thromboseartigen perimacularen Blutungen ist möglich.

IX. Conclusion

The manifold aspects of perinatal retinal haemorrhage have been discussed in each chapter. From the morphologic viewpoint, many new details were found through thorough histologic examination and comparison with fundus photographs. Even a detail of interest in general vessel pathology, hitherto overlooked or misinterpreted, was analyzed: the fibrin thrombus of vessel rupture. The discussion of macular haemorrhages and their sequelae was based on histologic findings; these demonstrate the likelihood that macular submembranacious haemorrhages hardly destroy any tissue.

In this book aetiologic factors influencing the incidence of haemorrhage are discussed. This discussion is based on the world literature, including very inaccessible papers. By means of this extensive survey, some tendencies were discovered because of the inclusion of rare courses of delivery.

Several questions remain open. It will always be difficult to clarify the individual anatomic and physiologic variations in the newborn, which seems to be responsible for the limited correlation of predisposing factors with retinal haemorrhage. More observations correlating the Apgar score to perinatal haemorrhage are desirable. Concerning the significance of retinal haemorrhages, more reexaminations after foveal involvement are necessary. Do perimacular haemorrhages influence the fusional amplitude? Can haemorrhages spread after birth? Is spontaneous fibrinolysis, an alteration occurring after birth, correlated with more extensive haemorrhages? Does the higher incidence of haemorrhage in infants born of primiparae depend on a prolonged second stage of labour? These are all questions that were not answered by our study.

Finally, it should be emphasized what an astonishing phenomenon perinatal retinal haemorrhage is! Birth, a physiologic process, causes spectacular alterations, namely vessel rupture and haemorrhage, in an extremely delicate organ, the retina. Even the functionally important macula is frequently affected. Regression begins after birth, and the alterations, comparable only to those in severe disease, are connected only with a brief episode of perinatal life.

X. Appendix

A. Plates

Some larger photographs to which the text refers on several occasions are collected in this appendix. The plates consist mainly of mosaic photographs of some interesting perinatal retinal haemorrhages. It should be kept in mind that only cases of particular interest were photographed, so that this is a selection of more severe cases. Some of them are compared to follow-up photographs. Two post mortem photographs of retinae are added to be compared with the in vivo photographs. One histologic section and a mosaic photograph of the fundus after fresh central venous occlusion are also included.

Plate I. Case I/50; mother: 15-year-old primipara; child: girl, birth weight 3250 g. Delivery: First stage of labour: 6 h 50 min; second stage: 28 min; vacuum extraction from left occipital presentation during prolonged second stage of labour.

a. **Right eye,** 24 h after birth: Several medium-sized haemorrhages at posterior pole, and one typical haemorrhage of nerve fibre layer with white fibrin thrombus in centre. Small submembranacious haemorrhage reaches macula. All haemorrhages absorbed within 1 week.

b. **Left eye,** 24 h after birth: Over 20 haemorrhages at posterior pole, linear and flame-shaped types, latter with typical white fibrin thrombi. Pear-shaped submembranacious haemorrhage originating from temporal inferior border of macula covers fovea. It originates from a flat haemorrhage, a white fibrin thrombus of which is visible as source of bleeding. Within 1 week, all flat haemorrhages absorbed, whereas submembranacious macular haemorrhage remained unaltered.

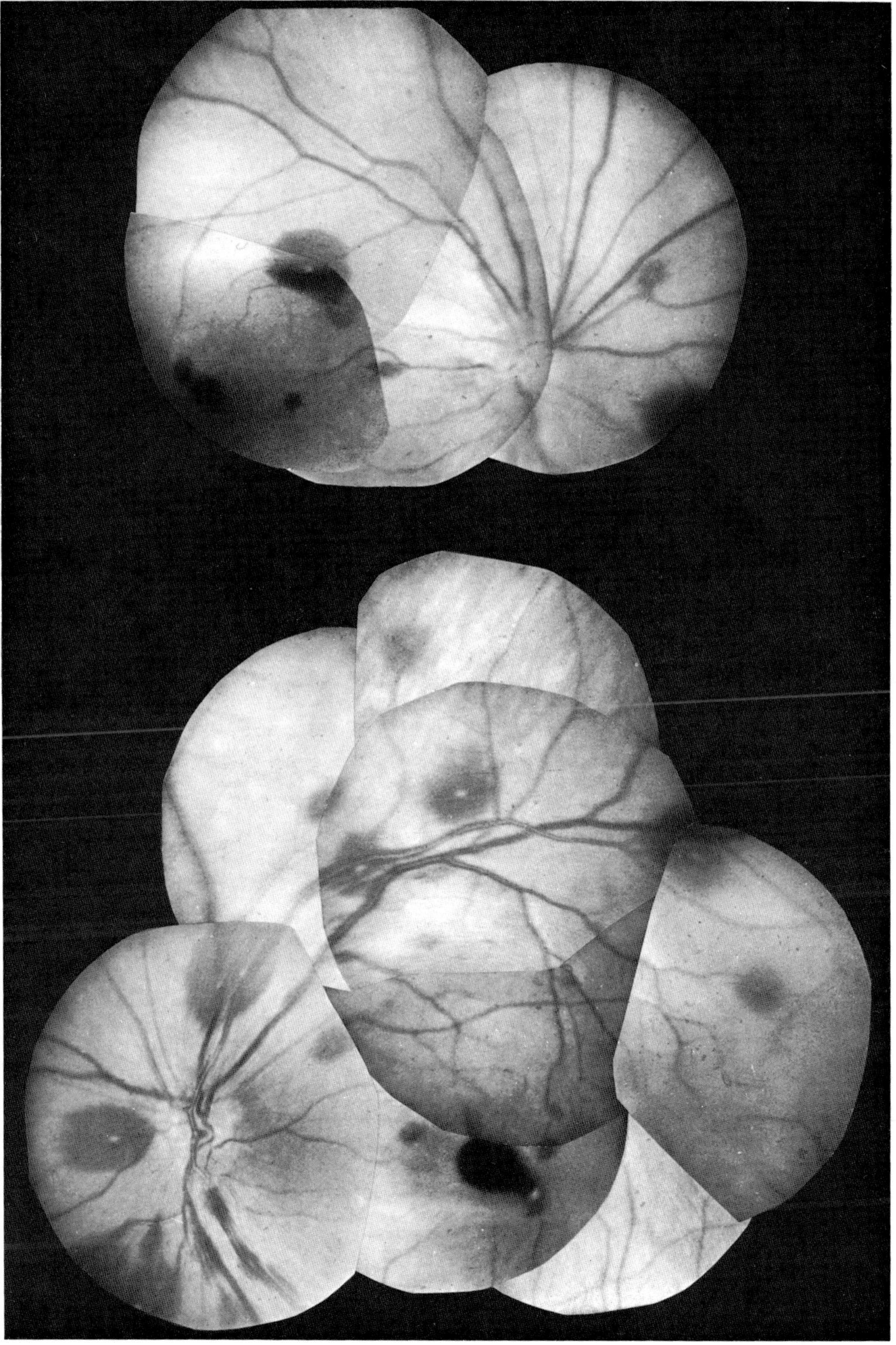

a
b

Plate II. Case III/34; mother: 25-year-old primipara; child: girl, birth weight 3000 g. Delivery: first stage of labour: 10 h 30 min; second stage: 15 min. Vacuum extraction from occipital presentation.

Right eye, 12 h after birth: Dispersed retinal haemorrhages around posterior pole and periphery. At clinical examination, number of haemorrhages estimated to be 10–20. Fundus photographs revealed that several linear haemorrhages had been overlooked. One haemorrhage of internal granular layer at macular border. Of special interest is a submembranacious haemorrhage in mid-periphery, with a typical white reflection on its centre. Within 5 days, all haemorrhages, including the submembranacious type, had been resorbed without visible sequelae.

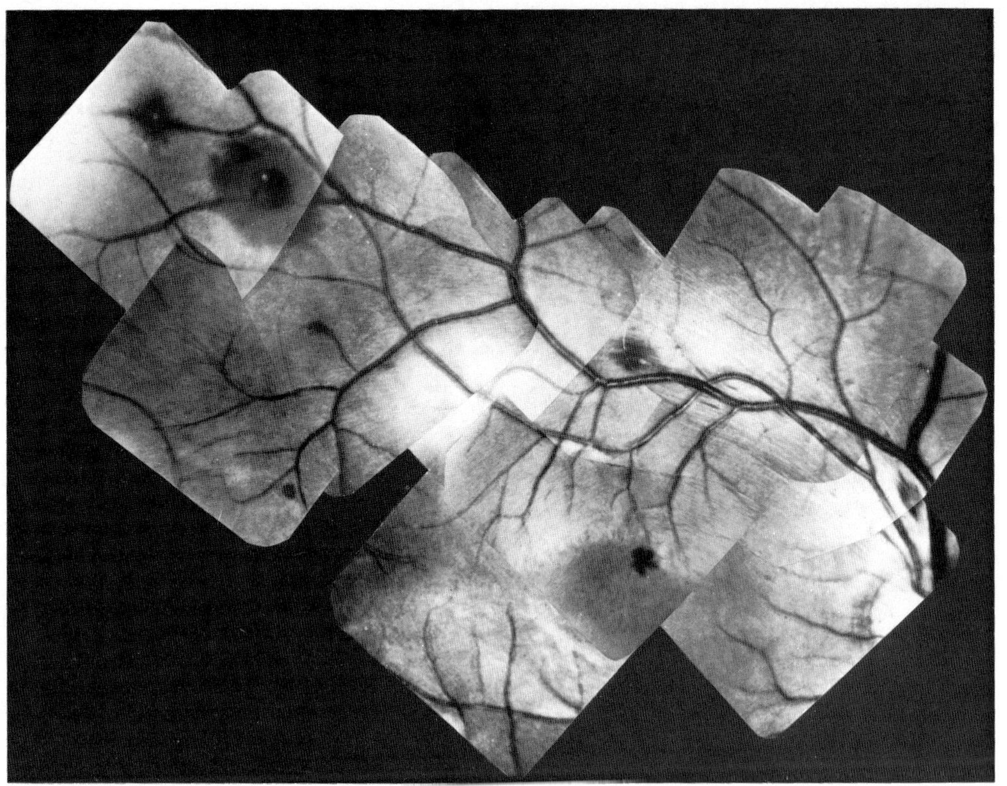

Plate III. Case III/34

Left eye, 12 h after birth: Multiple flat haemorrhages. Finest linear haemorrhages of nerve fibre layer prevail in area close to disc where this layer is particularly substantial. Flame-shaped type of nerve fibre layer haemorrhage extends to mid-periphery. Several granular haemorrhages of internal granular layer are clearly discernible because of dendritic outlines. Other less distinct haemorrhagic patches, as in upper nasal quadrant, must also be regarded as haemorrhages of granular layer, because of histologic findings. White centres at site of fibrin thrombi are also visible in several of the larger granular haemorrhages. No submembranacious haemorrhages, no macular involvement in this eye. After 5 days, only remnants of two haemorrhages at nasal and temporal side of macula still visible.

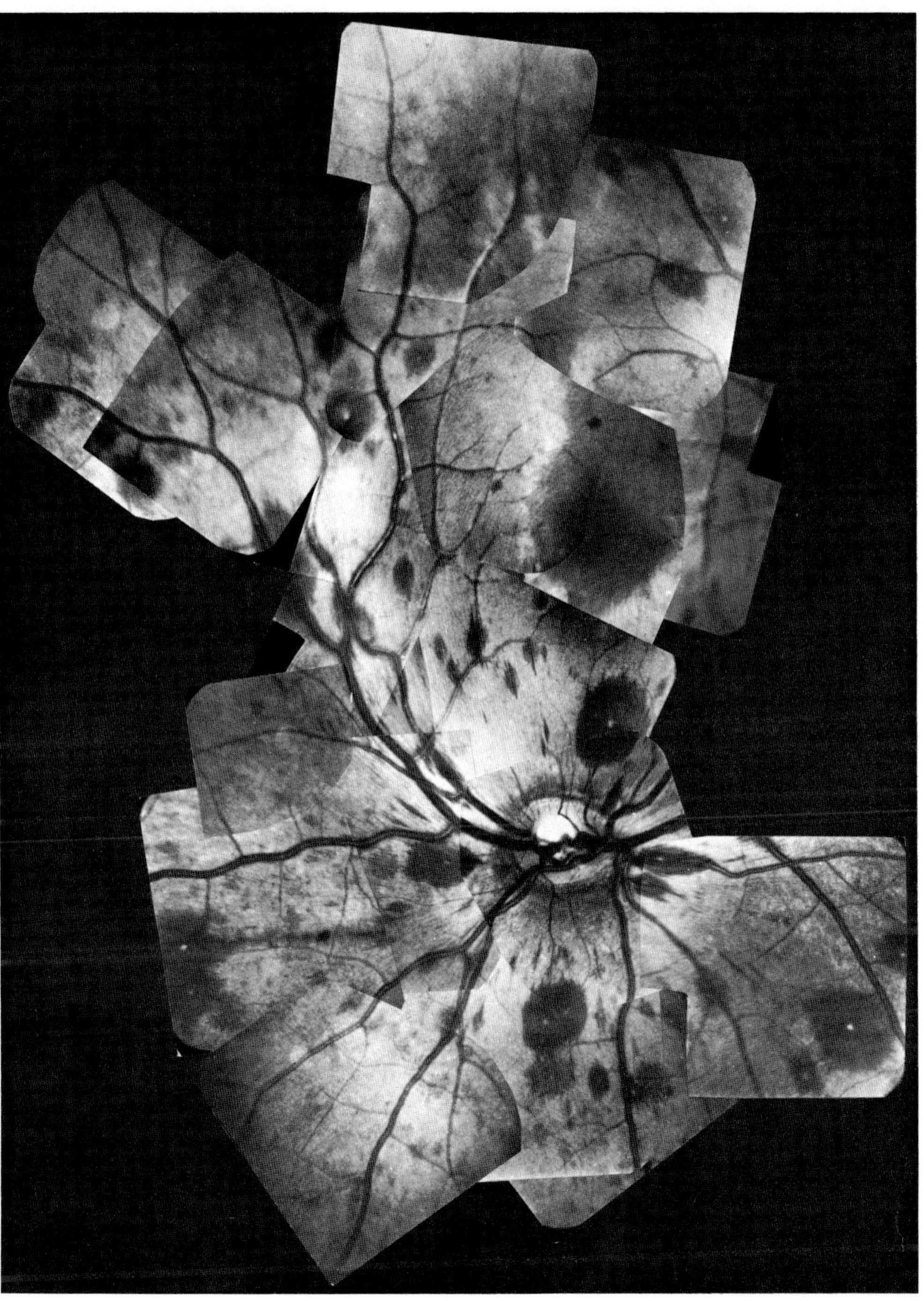

Plate IV. Case III/61; mother: 21-year-old primipara; child: girl, birth weight 3130 g. Delivery: first stage of labour: 7 h; second stage: 37 min. Pituitary preparation applied because of "inertia uteri". Spontaneous delivery from occipital presentation.

a. **Right eye**, 24 h after birth: A few haemorrhages only in the mid-periphery. One more extensive granular haemorrhage close to macular border. After 4 days, this had partly faded away but was still visible.

b. **Right eye**, follow-up at 5 years: No abnormalities visible at site of original haemorrhage.

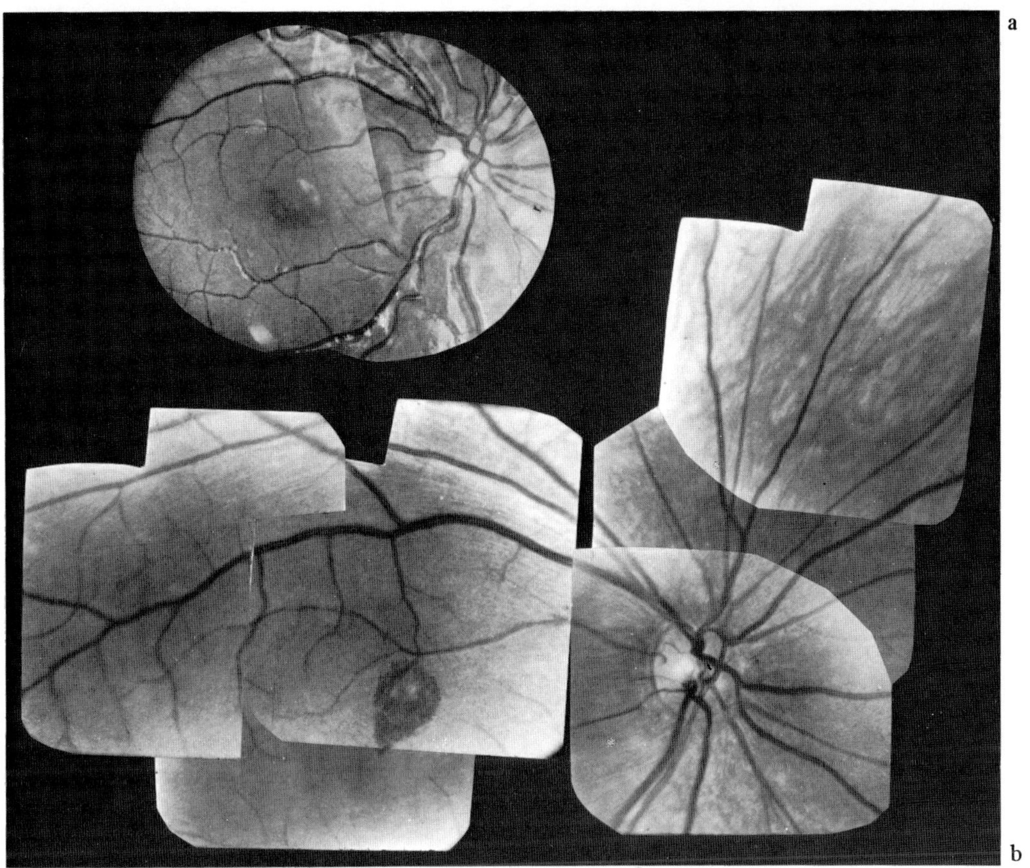

a
b

Plate V. Case III/61.

Left eye, 24 h after birth: Retinal haemorrhages at posterior pole and up to equatorial periphery. Haemorrhages of nerve fibre layer partly passing over border of disc, partly accompanying larger vessels. Outlines already slightly indistinct, due to incipient resorption. Granular haemorrhages seen especially in vicinity of macula. A single sub-membranacious haemorrhage covers macula. After 4 days, a few indistinct flat haemorrhages still visible. Macular haemorrhage unchanged (cf. Fig. 39 and follow-up, Fig. 63).

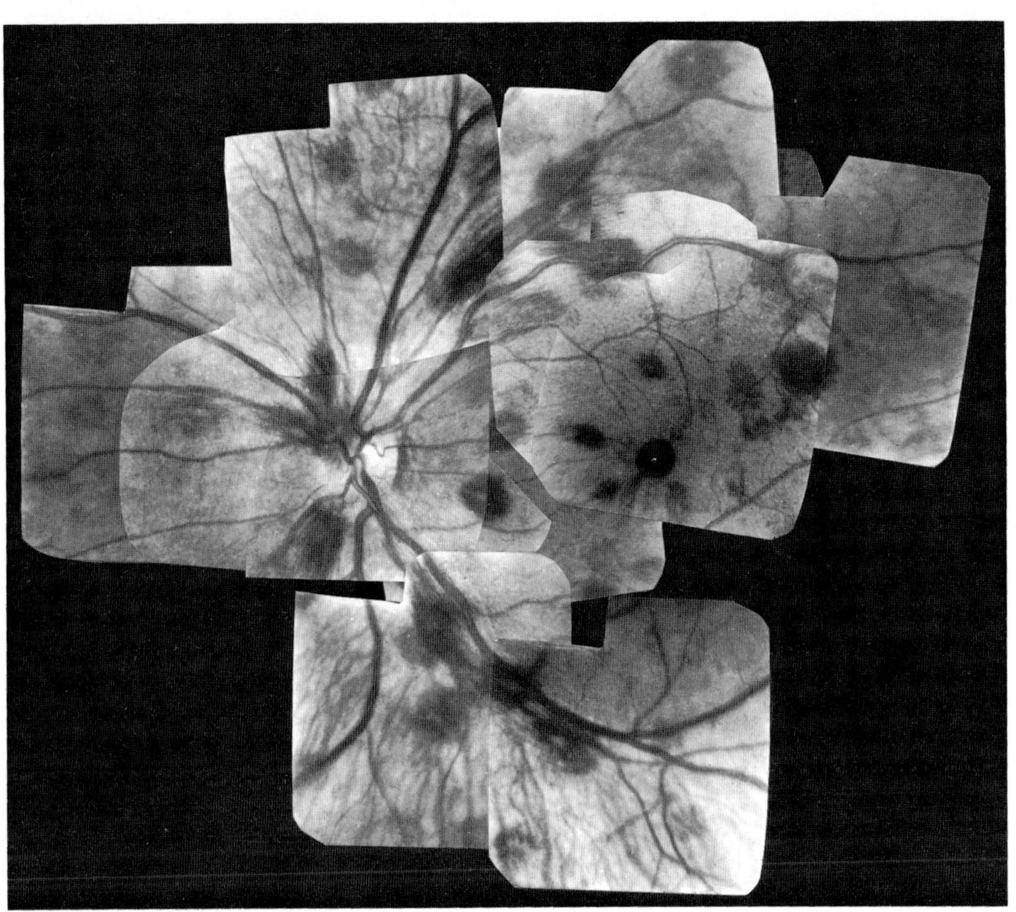

Plate VI. Case I/56, mother: 26-year-old primipara; child: boy, birth weight 3140 g. Delivery: first stage: 5 h, second stage: 10 min, spontaneous delivery from occipital presentation.

a. **Right eye**, 20 h after birth: Massive confluent haemorrhages, concentrated around posterior pole. Fundus photograph, technically imperfect, at least reveals multiple white fibrin thrombi of confluent flame-shaped haemorrhages of nerve fibre layer. Close to macula, three smaller submembranacious haemorrhages. One rather flat submembranacious haemorrhage touches macula from temporal inferior border. After 4 days, submembranacious haemorrhages still clearly visible. Number and distinctness of flat haemorrhages considerably altered.

b. **Right eye**, follow-up at age 6 years: Normal fundus, no irregularities corresponding to site of haemorrhages.

Fundus of left eye practically identical with one submembranacious haemorrhage reaching macula from 12 o'clock. At follow-up, visual acuity 1.0 o.u.; Titmus test: Rings Nos. 1—9 +; central fixation.

Plate VII. Case II/120; mother: 23-year-old primipara; child: boy, birth weight 3910 g. Delivery: first stage of labour: 3 h; second stage: 17 min. Vacuum extraction from first occipital presentation because of imminent asphyxia.

Left eye, 8 h after birth: Multiple, partly confluent flat haemorrhages from posterior pole to periphery. Multiple fibrin thrombi visible, especially in the haemorrhages of the nerve fibre layer. Several typical granular haemorrhages visible. Seven submembranacious haemorrhages in vicinity of disc and macular border; one of these covering macula and revealing its source by its peripheral white fibrin thrombus.

Right eye with similar involvement. After 6 days, practically all flat haemorrhages had vanished and all submembranacious haemorrhages were still visible.

VI

a

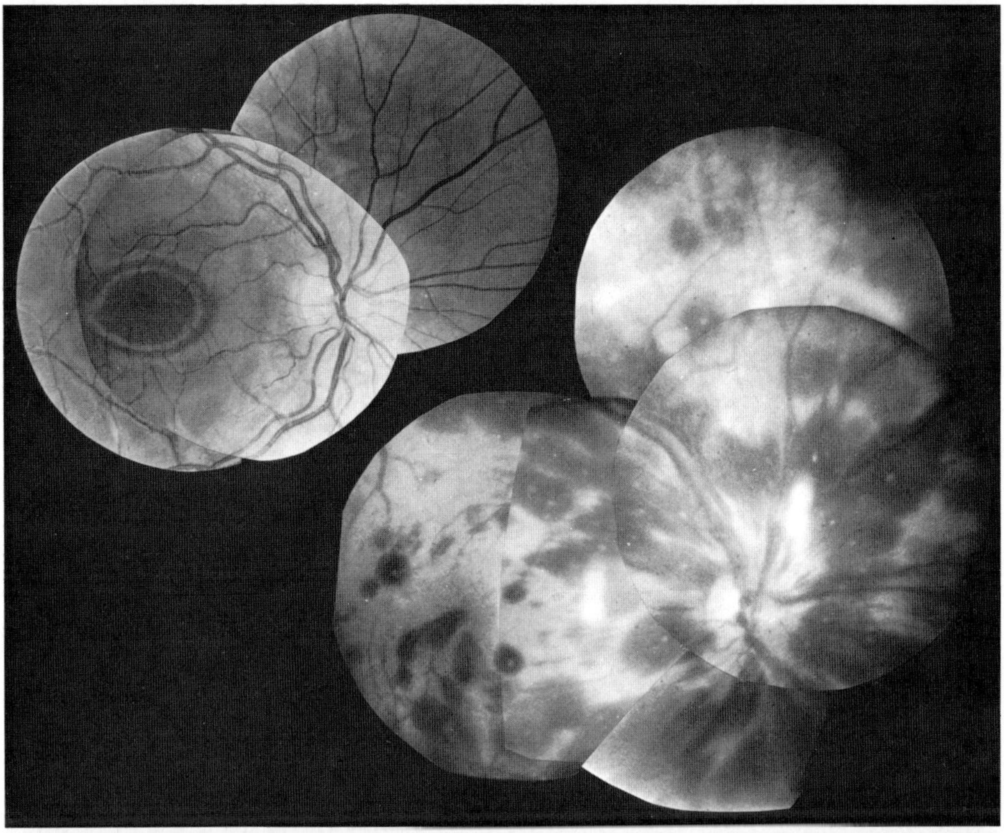

b

VII

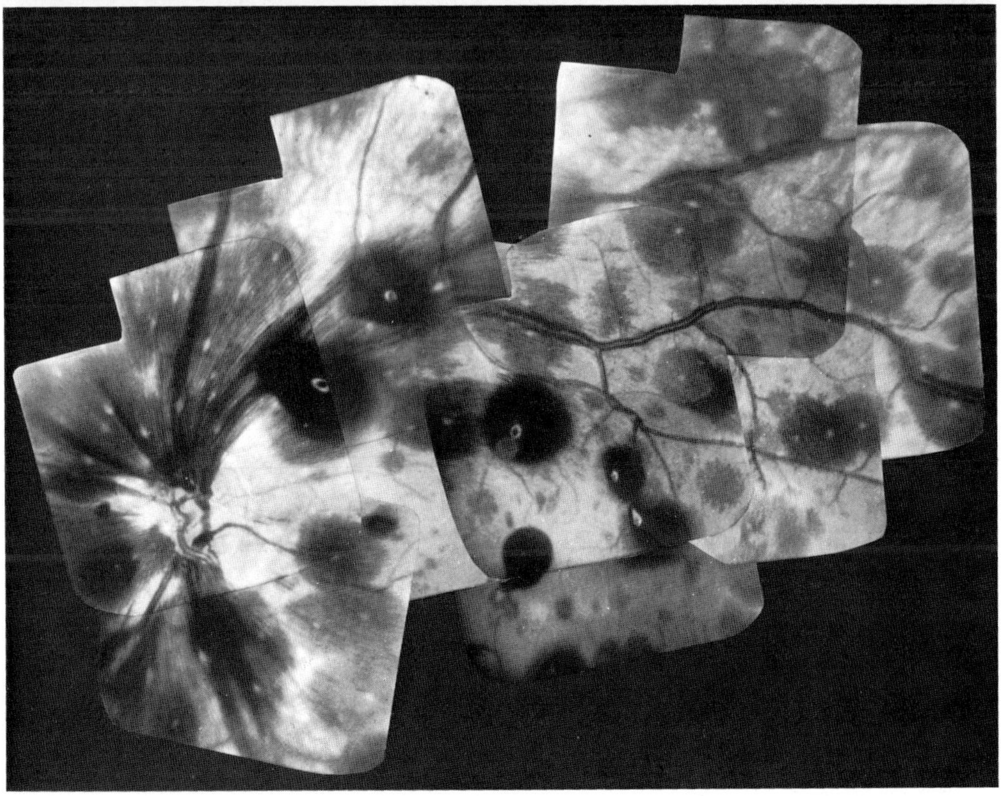

Plate VIII. Case III/31, mother: 33-year-old pluripara; child: girl, birth weight 3550 g. Delivery: First stage of labour: 5 h, second stage of labour: 4 min. Spontaneous delivery from occipital presentation.

a. **Right eye**, 6 h after birth: Close to disc retina is entirely invaded by confluent haemorrhages, studded with multiple white fibrin thrombi. Haemorrhages extend far into periphery. Typical granular and submembranacious haemorrhages are seen close to macula, sparing fovea.

b. **Right eye**, follow-up at age 6 years: Only single whitish depigmentation in midperiphery at 12 o'clock visible. Since no postnatal photographs correspond to this position, it remains unclear whether a particular type of haemorrhage at this area is the cause. At the site of other massive haemorrhages, no traces to be seen.

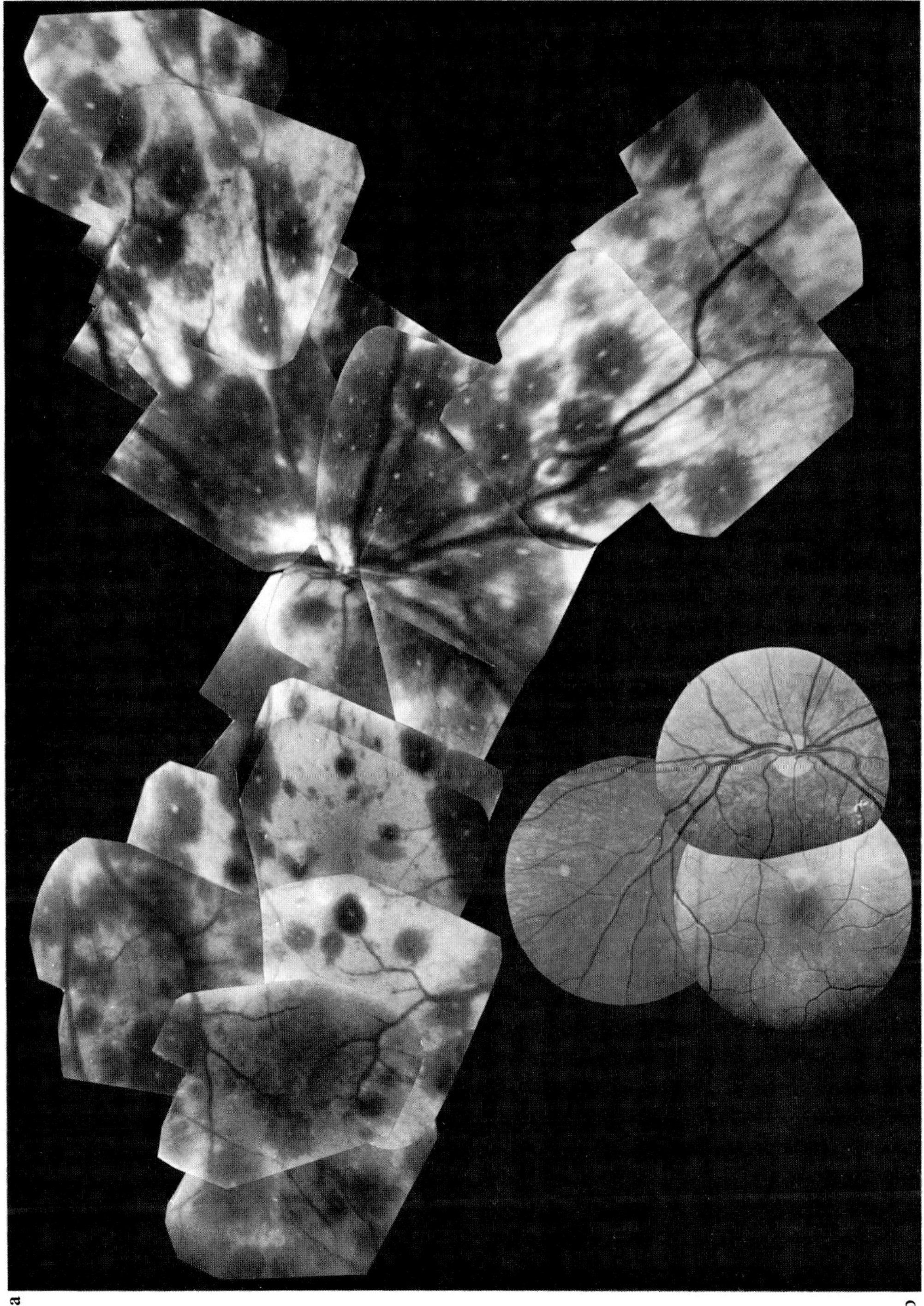
a
b

Plate IX. Case III/31.

a. **Left eye,** 6 h after birth: Multiple confluent haemorrhages of nerve fibre layer, especially along larger vessels, occupying major part of posterior pole. An important submembranacious haemorrhage in the shape of a calabash covers macula. After 8 days, all flat haemorrhages resorbed and the central submembranacious haemorrhage had concentrated to a hemisphere with circular outline, covering macula.

b. **Left eye,** follow-up at age 6 years: Normal fundus, no irregularities at site of former haemorrhages.

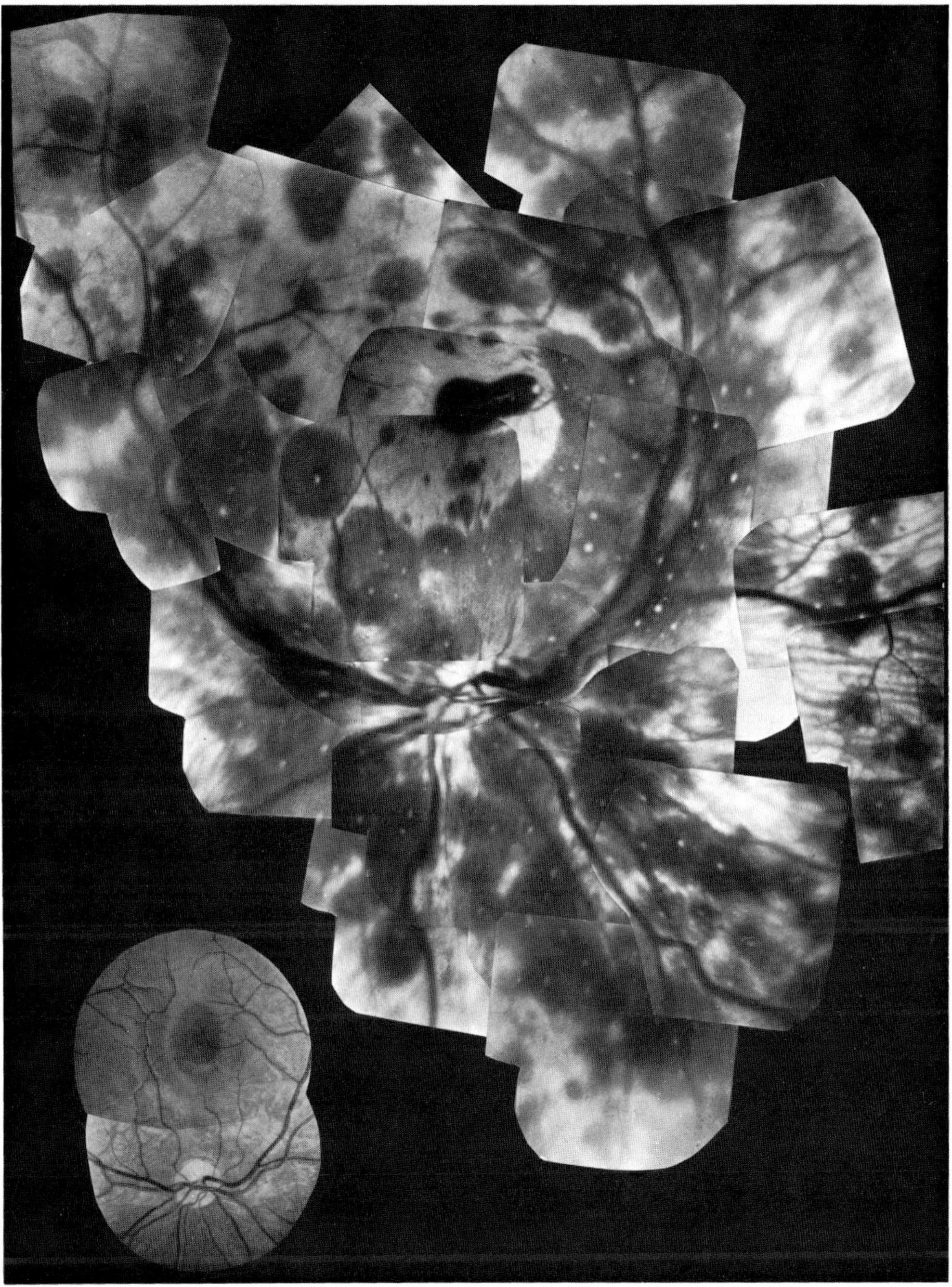
a
b

Plate X. Case III/28; mother 20-year-old secundipara; child: boy, birth weight 1810 g, immature. Multiple malformations of limbs. Forceps delivery because of imminent asphyxia. Died 2 h after birth.

Right eye: Partly fixed retina. Postmortal retinal folds at macula. The opaque retina makes haemorrhages particularly visible. Haemorrhages of nerve fibre layer can be seen in all dimensions, from single linear to confluent flame-shaped types with white fibrin thrombi. Granular haemorrhages are lighter in colour, most of them with a white centre. Where both haemorrhages overlap, histologically no communication was found. At the upper border, a large submembranacious haemorrhage hat not only detached the internal limiting membrane but also penetrated it, so that blood cells invaded the subhyaloid and the hyaloid space (cf. Fig. 54). The fusiform dilatation of a perivascular space, resembling a fusiform vessel dilatation, is visible at this same haemorrhage (cf. Fig. 18 and Plate XII).

Plate XI. Case III/28.

Left eye: A few haemorrhages in this eye, ranging from minute splinters to flames in the nerve fibre layer. Besides that, typical haemorrhages of the granular layer.

X

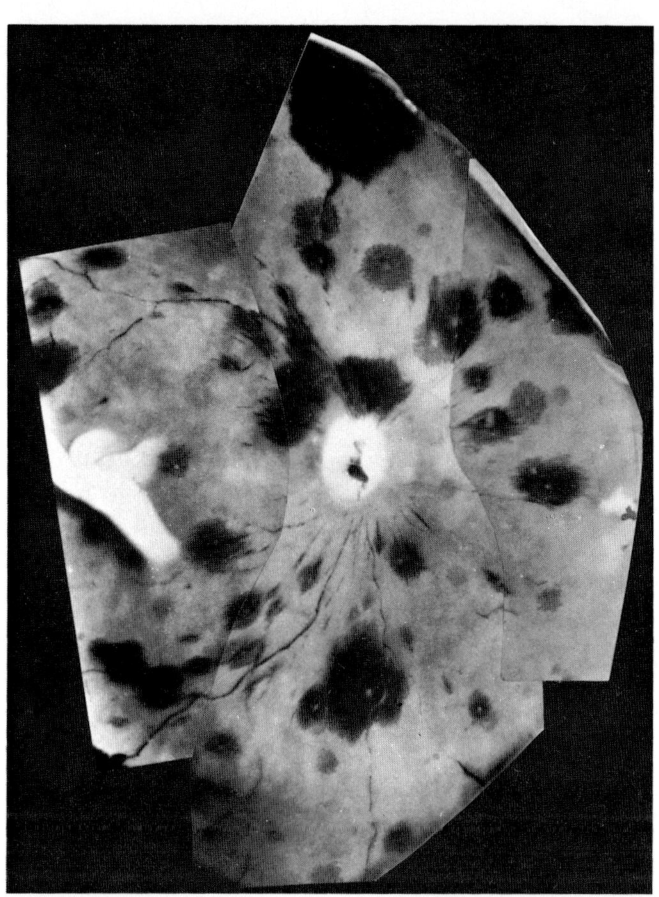

XI

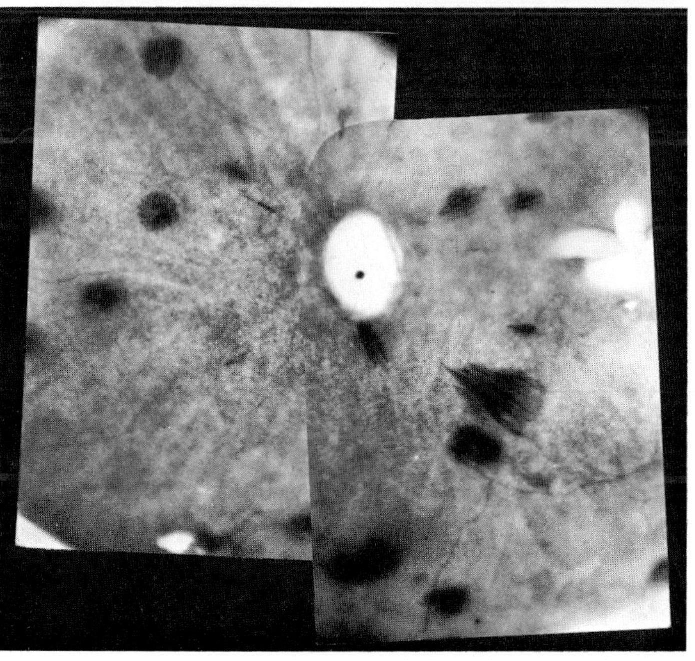

Plate XII. Section through confluent haemorrhage extending from ganglion cell layer to internal limiting membrane (central part of haemorrhage demonstrated in Plate X at superior border). To the right the eruption through the internal plexiform layer is visible, a section adjacent to Fig. 36. In the centre, in an arteriole, an intravital fibrin embolus stained darkly with PTAH. The embolus has no relation to the haemorrhage and its position is coincidental. To the left, the venule, also demonstrated in Fig. 18, is visible, with its perivascular space entirely invaded by blood cells.

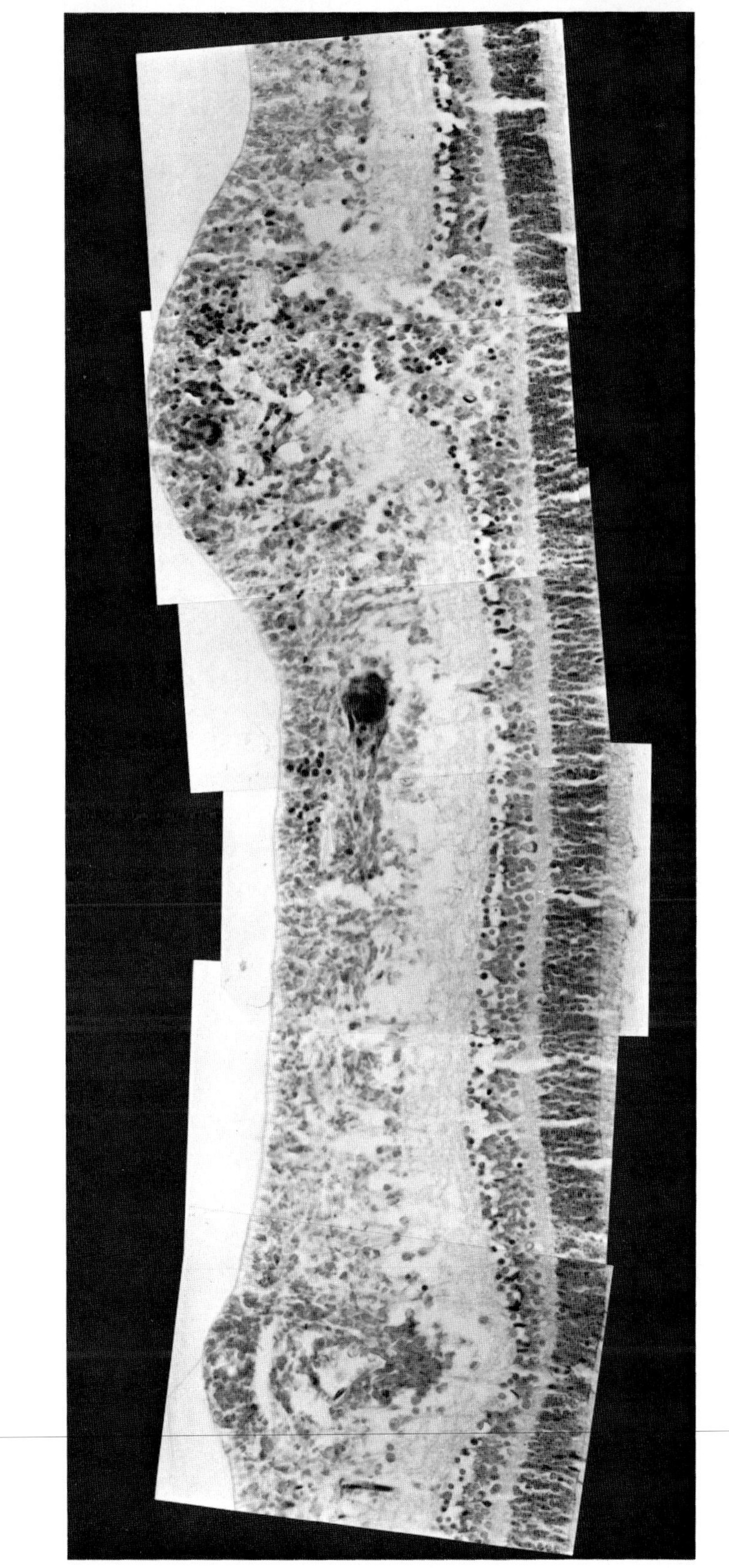

Plate XIII. 51-year-old patient with central venous occlusion of 2 days. Similar to perinatal haemorrhages here, also, extravasations are mainly situated at the posterior pole. Typical flame-shaped haemorrhages arranged along nerve fibres and with white centre visible. Granular haemorrhages, partly with clearly visible white centre, correspond to a certain extent to perinatal type. They differ because an orientation partly radial to macula, in accordance with tissue structures of Henle's layer. Thus, they partly cross the direction of the nerve fibres, which is not observed in perinatal haemorrhages.

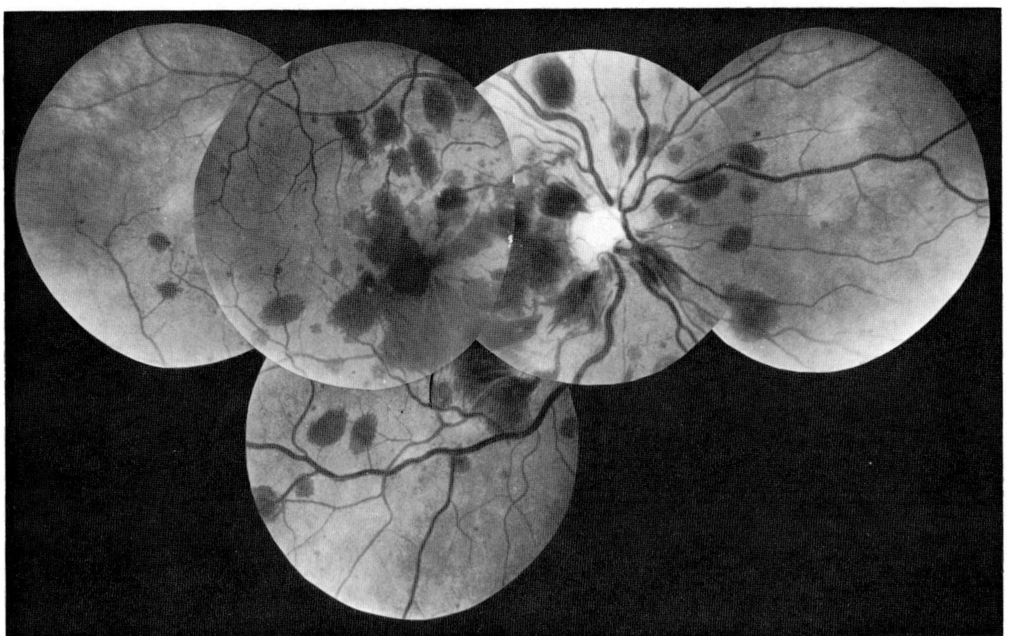

B. The First Description

Königstein's original text, the first description of perinatal retinal haemorrhage, is as
follows:

„Sehr häufig begegnet man verwaschenen rothen Flecken in verschiedener Größe
und Form. Ich konnte mir dieselben anfangs nicht deuten. Bei der Schwierigkeit, einzelne Punkte längere Zeit zu fixieren, konnte ich mir nicht Klarheit verschaffen, ob ich
es mit Extravasaten zu thun habe oder ob vielleicht an einer Stelle das Pigmentepithel
defect sei. Ich untersuchte mehrere solche Fälle nach einigen Tagen wieder, da war
aber keine Spur mehr jener Flecke zu sehen. Bei einem Kinde nun, das ich einige Stunden nach der Geburt untersuchte, sah ich in der Nähe der Papille zwei dunkelrote
Flecke von fast Papillengrösse, die ich ganz bestimmt als Blutextravasate ansprechen
konnte. Ich untersuchte nun das Kind täglich und bemerkte, wie die Extravasate
sowohl von der Peripherie als vom Centrum aus sich lichteten und so das verwaschene
Aussehen gewannen. Diese Beobachtung machte ich an mehreren Kindern. Hatte ich
Kinder aus den ersten Tagen, so waren die Flecken mehr oder weniger dunkelroth,
deutlich begrenzt, oft in den Glaskörper hineinragend, während Kinder aus den späte-
ren Tagen nur undeutliche verschwommene Flecken zeigten. Die Blutextravasate kom-
men nicht so selten vor; ich beobachtete sie in 10% meines Untersuchungsmaterials
und es wunderte mich darum, daß sie anderen Untersuchern entgangen sind. Sie sind
entweder radiär gestellt und streifenförmig die Gefäße begleitend oder in kleinen oder
größeren rundlichen Flecken, oft ist der ganze Augenhintergrund von innen bedeckt.
Wie schon oben angedeutet, werden sie rasch resorbirt und sind darum von keiner wei-
teren Bedeutung, doch könnte es immerhin möglich sein, daß durch massenhafte
Extravasate Retinaelemente zerstört werden, und sie dadurch Ursache später gefunde-
ner Amblyopien ohne Befund werden. Wann entstehen diese Extravasate und wodurch
werden sie hervorgerufen? Sicherlich entstehen sie nicht während des Uterinlebens.
Hiergegen spricht das Aussehen und die Analogie mit den Blutaustritten in die Haut
und die Conjunctiva. Sie können also nur während des Geburtsactes oder bei der durch
die ersten Athemzüge sich ändernden Blutcirculation entstehen. Für das Entstehen
während des Geburtsactes würde der große Druck, der allseitig auf das Kind ausgeübt
wird, sprechen, dagegen wäre zu erwähnen, daß bei schweren Zangengeburten, bei
Stirnlagen, bei sehr großen starken Kindern die Hämorrhagien relativ nicht häufiger
beobachtet werden, als bei kleinen Kindern, bei Frühgeburten, wo die Geburt eine
verhältnismäßig leichte und rasche ist. Meiner Ansicht nach liegt die Ursache in der
Circulationsänderung und Arterialisirung des Blutes. Ich hatte oft genug Gelegenheit
zu sehen, wie bei einem Kinde, das blau aussehend (venös) zur Welt kam, und das
sich nach mehreren Athemzügen rosa färbte, sich nun in der Haut zahlreiche Blutextravasate zeigten. Derselbe Vorgang findet wahrscheinlich auch in der Retina statt."

C. Bibliographic Notes

Goldwasser's paper (1914) contains the casuistics and literature of more than 100 titles, but only in the original "Dissertation", not in the version printed in *Beiträge zur Geburtshilfe und Gynäkologie.*

The paper by "M. Caurot" (1956, concours méd.) is only an excerpt from the paper by Edgar Cavrot (1956, Bruxelles med.).

The papers of the gynaecologist Koyama and of the ophthalmologists Yohitda, Yasuoka und Yoshida are based on the same series; the tables are more extensive in the ophthalmologic publication.

The Russian paper of Pushkash and Sabo is a shortened version of the Hungarian original of Puskás and Szabó. The notes about investigations by Frankowska and Przytula do not contain any details. The two papers by Jain and Gupta (1965) are practically identical. The two papers by Krauer-Mayer (1965) are also based on the same material. The survey is better in *Gynaecologica* (Basel).

The two titles of Vincenti and Gavinelli, published in the same year (1969) in *Minverva Ginecologica 21,* consist of an excerpt (pp. 426–427) and the complete paper (pp. 608–613).

Neme, Fraga, Salomao, Atzingen and Doneto-Santos published five subsequent articles, containing what would normally be different sections of the one article.

The denomination "perles jacobines" of Sourdille for submembranacious haemorrhages seemed to many bo be somewhat enigmatic. Since several French colleagues were unable to attach any significance to this term, one of these (Dr. Besnard) asked Dr. Sourdille directly and got the following answer (30.9.1971):

Je réponds à votre demande de rensignements concernant les "perles jacobines" découvertes au fond d'oeil dans les hématomes sous-duraux du nourrisson. Il s'agit de véritables petits hématomes pré-rétiniens sphériques, rappelant des perles de sang rouge noir.

L'épithète de "jacobin" se réfère aux aventures des dépouilles des rois de France enterrées dans la Basilique de Saint-Denis et qui furent exhumées et jetées à la rue lors de la Revolution de 1789. Par analogie abusive entre Jacobins, Terreur et sang versé, nous avions retenu l'expression de "perles jacobines" car cette description a été faite dans notre Service de l'Hôpital de Saint Denis.

Translated this reads:

In reply to your request for details on the "perles jacobines" observed in the fundus in subdural haematoma of babies: They are actually little preretinal, spheric haematomas, similar to beads of dark red blood.

The epithet "jacobin" refers to the adventures of sacking [the tombs of] the French kings buried in the Basilica of Saint-Denis. They were exhumed and thrown into the street during the revolution of 1789. Abusively alluding to the analogy between Jacobins, terror and bloodshed, we continued to use the expression "Perles Jacobines" because the description was coined in our department of the hospital of Saint-Denis.

Bibliography

Aliquò-Mazzei, A.: Le emorragie retiniche nei neonati. Attualità di ostetricia e ginecologica (Padova) *12*, 961–972 (1966)

Aron, J.J., Marx, P., Blanck, M.F., Duval, F., Luce, R.: Signes oculaires observés dans le syndrome de Silverman. Ann. Oculist. *203*, 533–546 (1970)

Arruga, A.: Examen ocular en el recién nacido. Rec. Españ. Pediat. *11*, 453–459 (1955)

Aurand, L.: Scotome central méconnu, par rétinite proliférante papillomaculaire consécutive à des hémorrhagies rétiniennes d'origine obstétricale. Bull. Soc. Ophthalmol. Fr.   , 615–622 (1939)

Aust, W., Kirsch, D., Herrmann, E.: Glaskörper- und Fundusveränderungen bei akuten Subarachnoidalblutungen. Ber. Dtsch. Ophthalmol. Ges. *68*, 75–79 (1967)

Azevedo, G. de, Ribeiro, A., Moreira, M.: O Exame do fundo do olho em récem-nascido de parto espontâneo e de parto com ventosa. Rev. Clin. Inst. Matern. (Lisboa) 45–47 (1963)

Bachmann, K.D., Friedmann, G., Weiden, H., Springmann, L., Schmidt, E., Bolte, A.: Pathologische Befunde bei Neugeborenen nach Entbindung durch Vakuumextraktion (Netzhautblutungen, Schädelfrakturen, EEG-Veränderungen). Geburtshilfe Frauenheilkd. *28*, 1089–1103 (1968)

Bahn, C.A.: Discussion of Signorelli. New Orleans Md. Surg. J. *79*, 454 (1926)

Baillart, P.: Affections vasculaires de la rétine. Paris: G. Doin 1953

Ballantyne, A.J.: The ocular manifestations of spontaneous subarachnoid haemorrhage. Br. J. Ophthalmol. *27*, 383–414 (1943)

Barsewisch, B. von: Die Netzhautblutungen des Neugeborenen, Morphologie, Ätiologie, Bedeutung. Habilitationsschrift: Ludwig-Maximilians-Universität München 1972, 335 p.

Barsewisch, B. von: Über Kreislauffaktoren bei perinatalen Fundusblutungen. Klin. Monatsbl. Augenheilkd. *167*, 772–773 (1975)

Barsewisch, B. von, Hickl, E.-J.: Retinablutungen bei Neugeborenen. Vortrag, Tagung der Vereinigung Bayerischer Augenärzte, München 9.–10.5.1970. Summary: Klin. Monatsbl. Augenheilkd. *159*, 121 (1971)

Baum, J.D.: Retinal photography in premature infants: Forme fruste retrolental fibroplasia. Proc. R. Soc. Med. *64*, 777–779 (1971)

Baum, J.D., Bulpitt, C.J.: Retinal and conjunctival haemorrhage in the newborn. Arch. Dis. Child. *45*, 344–349 (1970)

Bedell, A.J.: Discussion of: Jacobs, M.W.: Retinal hemorrhage in the newborn. J. Am. Med. Assoc. *83*, 1644–1645 (1924)

Belmonte, N.: Discussion of: Orduña, G., De Arizcun Pineda, J.: El fondo de ojo como indice de valoración de las diferentes tecnicas de parto. Arch. Soc. Oftalmol. Hisp.-Amer. *30*, 276 (1970)

Belmonte Gonzales, J.: Hemorragias retinianas del recién nacido. Rev. Esp. Otoneurooftalmol. Neurocir. *6*, 323; 393–408 (1947)

Bergen, R., Margolis, S.: Retinal hemorrhages in the newborn. Ann. Ophthalmol. *8*, 53–56 (1976)

Berger, E.: Les maladies des yeux dans leurs rapports avec la pathologie générale. Paris: Masson 1892, 205 pp.

Berger, E., Loewy, R.: Über Augenerkrankungen sexuellen Ursprungs bei Frauen. Wiesbaden: Bergmann 1906, pp. 116–119

Birich, T.V., Peretitskaya, V.N.: Organ of vision in children with retinal hemorrhage sustained in the neonatal period. Vestn. Oftalmol. *4*, 23–37 (1968)

Blanc, B.: Le fond d'oeil du nouveau-né. Presse Méd. *75*, 347–348 (1967)

Bleyl, U., Büsing, C.M.: Kreislaufschock und disseminierte intravasale Gerinnung bei intrauterinem und perinatalem Fruchttod. Klin. Wochenschr. *48*, 13–24 (1970)

Bonamour, M.: Discussion of: Aurand. L.: Scotome central méconnu, par retinite proliferante papillo-maculaire consécutive à des hémorragies rétiniennes d'origine obstétricale. Bull. Soc. Ophthalmol. Fr. 621 (1939)

Bonamour, M.G.: Le prognostic éloigné des hémorrhagies rétiniennes du nouveau-né. Bull. Mém. Soc. Fr. Ophthalmol. *62*, 227–236 (1949)

Bousquet, F.P., Laupus, W.E.: Studies on the pathogenesis of retrolental fibroplasia. Am. J. Ophthalmol. *35*, 64–68 (1952)

Braendstrup, P.: Ophthalmological experiences in a paediatric department. Acta Ophthalmol. *32*, 729–733 (1954)

Braendstrup, P.: Vitreous haemorrhage in the newborn. A rare type of neonatal intra-ocular haemorrhage. Acta Opthalmol. *47*, 502–513 (1969)

Brogi, M., Del Buono, G., Pandolfi, M.: Le emorragie retiniche del neonato. Ann. Ottalmol. *88*, 657–674 (1962)

Brückner, R., Bloch, W., Wolff-Wiesinger, L.: Zur Genese der Retina- und Opticus-Scheidenblutungen bei akuter intrakranieller Drucksteigerung. Ophthalmologica *118*, 607–610 (1949)

Bruniquel, G., Dollard, H.: Épreuve double-aveugle sur les hémorrhagies rétiniennes du nouveau-né: resultats en contradiction formelle avec certaine statistique alarmante après vacuum-extractor. Bull. Féd. Gynécol. Obstét. Fr. *20*, 296–298 (1968)

Buchanan, L.: Discussion on birth injuries of the eye, opening paper. Trans. Ophthalmol. Soc. U.K. *46*, 32–42 (1926)

Buchhalter, I., Schnecke, D.: Beitrag zur Problematik der Fundusblutungen bei Neugeborenen. Sitzung der Berliner Augenärztl. Ges., Dez. 1967. Klin. Monatsbl. Augenheilkd. *153*, 133 (1968)

Bulpitt, C.J., Baum, J.D.: Retinal photography in the newborn. Arch. Dis. Child. *44*, 499–503 (1969)

Burian, H.M.: Discussion of: Enoch, J.M.: Receptor amblyopia. Am. J. Ophthalmol. *48*/II, 262–274 (1959)

Caffey, J.: The whiplash shaken infant syndrome: Manual shaking by the extremities with whiplash-induced intracranial and intra-ocular bleedings, linked with residual permanent brain damage and mental retardation. Pediatrics *54*, 397–403 (1974)

Calmettes, L., Deodati, F., Bec, P.: Étude histo-pathologique de la chorio-rétine des prématurés. Doc. Ophthalmol. *20*, 420–440 (1966)

Candian, B.: Il fondo oculare del neonato. Rass. Ital. Ottalmol. *18*, 3–16 (1949)

Canon, R., Guilhem, P., Mayer, M.: L'anoxie foetale. XVe Congrès Féd. Soc. Gynécol. Obstét. Fr., Alger-Tunis, 1952. Bull. Fed. Soc. Gynecol. Obstet. Fr. *4*/1, 145–242 (1953)

Capper, A.: The fate and development of the immature and of the premature child. Am. J. Dis. Child. *35*, 262–288; 443–491 (1928)

Casanovas, J., Torres Marty, L., Marín, M.: Observaciones sobre las hemorragias retinianas y otras alteraciones oftalmológicas en los recién nacidos. Arch. Padiatr. (Barcelona) *9*, 605–616 (1959)

Castrén, J.A.: Pathogenesis and treatment of Terson-Syndrome. Acta Ophthalmol. (Kbh.) *41*, 430–434 (1963)

Cavrot, E.: À propos des hémorragies rétiniennes du nouveau-né à terme. Brux. Méd. *36*, 514–520; 555–563 (1956)

Cavrot, E., Humblet, M., Richard, J.: L'hémorragie rétinienne du nouveau-né à terme. Ses rapports avec la fragilité vasculaire du nouveau-né et l'hémorragie cérébro-méningée. Essai de prophylaxie. Arch. Fr. Pediatr. *12*, 1085–1106 (1955)

Chang, J.M.: Newborn retinal hemorrhage and amblyopia. Trans. Ophthalmol. Soc. Rep. China *13*, 21–25 (1974)

Chase, R.R., Merritt, K.K., Bellows, M.: Ocular findings in the newborn infant. A.M.A. Arch. Opthalmol. *44*, 236–242 (1950)

Chosson, J., et al.: Considerations sur l'étude du fond d'oeil du nouveau-né. Rev. Fr. Gynécol. *62*, 703–709 (1967)

Cibis, P.A.: Vitreoretinal pathology and surgery in retinal detachment. St. Louis: C.V. Mosby 1965

Ciechanowska, A., Bryniak, C., Przepiórkowski, R., Markowska-Kraik, E.: Retinal hemorrhages in newborns. Przegl. Lek. *31*, 838–842 (1974)

Coburn, E.B.: Hemorrhages in the eye, present at birth. Arch. Ophthalmol. *33*, 256–267 (1904)

Cook, R.C., Glascock, R.E.: Refractive and ocular findings in the newborn. Am. J. Ophthalmol. *34*, 1407–1413 (1951)

Cordero Moreno, R., Najul, Y.: Estudio del fondo de ojo en el recién nacido. Arch. Ven. Puericultura Pediatría *21*, 285–295 (1958)

Cramer, E.: Verletzungen und Berufskrankheiten des Auges. In: Kurzes Handbuch der Ophthalmologie. Schieck, F., Brückner, A. (eds.), Vol. 4. Berlin: Springer 1931

Crehange, J.: L'examen du fond d'oeil du nouveau-né normal. Paris: Thèse 1958, 56 pp.

Critchley, E.M.R.: Observations on retinal haemorrhages in the newborn. J. Neurol. Neurosurg. Psychiatry (London) *31*, 259–262 (1968)

Croci, C., Scardaccione, M.: Le emorragie retiniche dei neonati. Boll. Ocul. *19*, 877–917 (1940)

Croci, C., Scardaccione, M.: Sugli esiti a distanza delle emorragie retiniche dei neonati. Boll. Ocul. *20*, 836–846 (1941)

Cushing, H., Bordley, J.: Observations on experimentally induced choked disc. Johns Hopkins Med. J. *20*, 95–101 (1909)

Digonnet, L., Chan, J., Pierre, R.: Nouvelles études sur la résistance capillaire du nouveau-né et de la femme au cours du travail. Bull. Féd. Soc. Gynecol. Obstet. Fr. *4/1*, 649–655 (1952)

Dixon, J.M., Paul, E.V.: Separation of the pars ciliaris retinae in retrolental fibroplasia. Am. J. Ophthalmol. *34*, 182–190 (1951)

Doege, E.: Über die Histologie der Fundusblutungen bei Neugeborenen. Wissenschaftl. Z. Univ. Rostòck *18*, M 9/10, Teil I, 1075–1078 (1969)

Doggart, J.H.: Diseases of children's eyes. London: H. Kimpton 1950

Dolcet-Buxeres, L., Ferrer-Pi, S.: Hemorrhagias retinianas del recién nacido. Arch. Pediatr. (Barcelona) *5*, 1–8 (1954)

Dorello, U., Poli, L.: L'aspetto oftalmoscopico del fundus nel neonato prematuro. Arch. Ottalmol. *17*, 17–23 (1953)

Döring, G.K., Krauß, V.: Über die Bedeutung der Geburtsdauer für das Kind. Geburtshilfe Frauenheilkd. *27*, 1185–1193 (1967)

Douglas, A.A.: Children of reduced birth weight. Clin. Develop. Med. *32*, 82–86 (1969)

Dowling, J.E., Boycott, B.B.: Neural connections of the primate retina. Eye Structure, II. Symp. Rohen, J.W. (ed.). Stuttgart: Schattauer 1965, pp. 55–68

Drews, L.C., Minckler, J.: Massive bilateral pre-retinal hemorrhage. Am. J. Ophthalmol. *27*, 1–15 (1944)

Drozdova, M.V.: About particular observations of the normal fundus and about retinal haemorrhages in the newborn. Vestn. Oftalmol. *30*, 20–23 (1951)

Duesberg, H., Tiburtius, H.: Über Netzhautblutungen bei Neugeborenen. Zentralbl. Gynäkol. *80*, 1561–1565 (1958)

Duhard, J.-P., Pages, D.: Bilan oculaire systématique chez le nouveau-né. Appreciation de son intérêt à partir d'une étude en serie continue de 150 cas. Presse Méd. *2*, 2275–2276 (1973)

Duke Elder, Sir St. (ed.): System of Ophthalmology Vol. II, The anatomy of the visual system. London: H. Kimpton 1961

Duke Elder, Sir St. (ed.): System of ophthalmology. Vol. X; Diseases of the retina.
    Duke Elder, Sir St., Dobree, J.H. London: H. Kimpton 1967, p. 137
Duke Elder, Sir St. (ed.): System of ophthalmology. Vol. XII, Neuroophthalmology.
    Haemorrhage into the optic nerve sheaths. London: H. Kimpton 1971, p. 26
Dyer, N., Raye, J., Gutberlet, R., Faxelius, G., Swanstrom, S., Brill, A., Stahlman, M.:
    Timing of intracranial bleeding in newborn infants. Annual Meeting European Soc.
    for Paediatric Research, Brighton, 22.–26. June 1971
Eades, M.F.: Retinal haemorrhages of the newborn. N. Engl. Med. 201, 151–155 (1929)
Edgerton, A.E.: Ocular observations and studies of the newborn. A.M.A. Arch. Oph-
    thalmol. 11, 838–867 (1934)
Ehlers, N., Jensen, J.K., Hansen, K.B.: Retinal haemorrhages in the newborn. Compari-
    son of delivery by forceps and by vacuum extraction. Acta Ophthalmol. 52, 73–82
    (1974)
Ehrenfest, H.: Birth injuries of the child. New York–London: D. Aplleton 1922
Ely, E.T.: Ophthalmoscopic observations upon the refraction of the eyes of newly-
    born children. Arch. Opthalmol. 9, 29–40 (1880). Translated: Beobachtungen mit
    dem Augenspiegel bezüglich der Refraktion Neugeborener. Arch. Augenheilkd. 9,
    431–422 (1880)
Evelbauer, K.: Der Vakuumextraktor im praktisch-klinischen Gebrauch. Geburtshilfe
    Frauenheilkd. 3, 223–230 (1956)
Evelbauer, K.: Vakuum-Extraktion. Arch. Gynäkol. 198, 523–543 (1963)
Evsyokova, I.I., Reinish, M.S.: Genesis of retinal hemorrhages in neonates. Vopr. Okhr.
    Materin Det. 14, 61–65 (1969)
Evsyukova, I.E.: Retinal hemorrhages in newborn infants. Vopr. Okhr. Materin Det.
    14, 87 (1969)
Fahmy, J.A.: Symptoms and signs of intracranial aneurysms, with particular reference
    to retinal haemorrhage. Acta Ophthalmol. 50, 129–136 (1972a)
Fahmy, J.A.: Vitreous haemorrhage in subarachnoid haemorrhage – Terson's syn-
    drome. Acta Ophthalmol. 50, 137–143 (1972b)
Fahmy, J.A.: Fundal haemorrhages in ruptured intracranial aneurysms. II. Correlation
    with the clinical course. Acta Ophthalmol. 51, 299–304 (1973)
Falls, H.F., Jurow, H.N.: Effect on antepartum vitamin K on retinal hemorrhage. J.
    Am. Med. Assoc. 131, 203–205 (1946)
Ferreira, L.E.: O examine de fundo de ôlho nos prematuros. Arq. Brasil. Oftalmol. 18,
    185–195 (1955)
Figueroa, M.: Contribución al estudio de la hemorragia retinal del recién nacido. Arch.
    Chil. Opftalmol. 15, 101 (1958)
Fine, B.S., Yanoff, M.: Ocular histology. New York: Harper and Row 1972, 260 p.
Fontaine, M.: Manifestations oculaires de la prématurité. Arch. Ophthalmol. Fr. 31,
    383–388 (1971)
Foster Moore, R.: Discussion on the significance of retinal haemorrhages. Br. Med. J.
    2, 1097–1101 (1926)
Franceschetti, A., Balavoine, C.: Considerazioni oftalmologiche sulle emorragie del
    neonato. Atti del XXI Congresso della Società Italiana di Pediatria, Venezia, 16.–
    19. Sept. 1951, reprint, 5 pp.
Franceschetti, A.: Round table session I. In: International Strabismus Symposium.
    Arruga, A. (ed.). Basel–New York: Karger 1968, pp. 78–79
François, J., Neetens, A.: The blood-supply of the optic nerve. Eye structure. II. Symp.
    Rohen, J.W. (ed.). Stuttgart: Schattauer 1965, pp. 187–203
François, J., Tranos, L.: L'étiologie des hémorrhagies oculaires chez le nouveau-né.
    Ann. Oculist. 208, 185–196 (1975)
Frankowska, J., Przytula, P.: Intraocular haemorrhages of the newborn and their rela-
    tion to birth trauma. Congr. Oculist. (Polska) 1, 126 (1954)
Freitas, J.A.M. de: Hemorragia retiniana no recém-nascido. Rev. Pesq. Med. (Fortaleza)
    3, 5–8 (1965)

Freitas, J.A.H. de, Garcia, F.N.: O estudio do fondo do olhô em recém-nascidos. Rev. Bras. Oftalmol. *27*, 199–225 (1968)

Fritz, A., Parent, G., Lambilliotte, A., Beeckman, G.: Physiopathologie des hémorragies rétiniennes obstétricales. Bull. Soc. Belge Ophthalmol. *142*, 475–489 (1966)

Fuchs, E.: Lehrbuch der Augenheilkunde, 10. ed. Leipzig–Wien: F. Deuticke 1905

Fulst, W.: Über Einwirkungen des Vakuumextraktors am kindlichen Schädel und Gehirn. Zentralbl. Gynäkol. *82*, 321–328 (1960)

Fung, M.S., Young, M.F., Chang, J.M.: Retinal hemorrhage in the newborn. Trans. Soc. Ophthalmol. Sin. *7*, 51–62 (1968); Ophthalmol. Lit. (London) *22*, 432 (1968) (excerpt)

Gajaria, A.T., Abreu, A.T., Gokhale, S.N.: Incidence of haemorrhages in the newborn. I. Normal deliveries. J. All-India Ophthalmol. Soc. *13*, 43–49 (1965)

Gärtner, J.: Histologische Beobachtungen über die Struktur der vitreoretinalen Grenzschicht. (Zur Frage der Existenz von M. hyaloidea and M. limitans interna retinae). Klin. Monatsbl. Augenheilkd. *141*, 261–280 (1962)

Gärtner, J.: Die Feinstruktur der Glaskörperrinde des menschlichen Auges an der Ora serrata im Alter. Graefes Arch. Ophthalmol. *168*, 529–562 (1965)

Giles, C.L.: Retinal haemorrhages in the newborn. Am. J. Ophthalmol. *49*, 1005–1011 (1960)

Glavanakova, V., Valov, V., Georgieva, L.: Retinal haemorrhages in the newborn. Akush. Ginek. Sofiya *7*, 356–358 (1968); Ophthalmol. Lit. (London) *22*, 683 (1968) (exerpt)

Goldwasser, J.: Über die Augenverletzungen bei der Geburt und besonders bei der Zangenoperation und ihre gerichtlich-medizinische Bedeutung. Leipzig: Inaugural-Disseration, Universität München 1914, 60 p. (excerpt: Beitr. Geburtshilfe Gynäkol. *19*, 365–405 (1914)

Gombos, G.M., Schenker, J.G.: Retinal hemorrhage in the newborn after complicated delivery. Harefuah *72*, 299–300 (1967)

Göttinger, W.: Intraokulare Blutung bei einer Hirnmassenblutung. Klin. Monatsbl. Augenheilkd. *159*, 819–823 (1971)

Gottstein, I., Schnecke, D.: Ergebnisse der Nachuntersuchungen bei Kindern mit Fundusblutungen post natum. Klin. Monatsbl. Augenheilkd. *162*, 119 (1973)

Grassi, L., Musini, A.: Contributo allo studio dell'etiologia e della patogenesi delle emorragie retiniche dei neonati. Sangue (Milano) *23*, 157–163 (1950)

Greear, J.N.: Rupture of aneurysm of the circle of Willis. Relationship between intraocular and intra-cranial hemorrhage. A.M.A. Arch. Ophthalmol. *30*, 312–319 (1943)

Grigera, E.J.: Hemorragias oculares en el recién nacido. Arch. Oftalmol. (B. Aires) *39*, 318–322 (1964)

Groot, V.M. de, Friedenwald, J.S.: Thrombi in the ciliary veins of eyes from newborn infants. Am. J. Ophthalmol. *43*, 93–96 (1957)

Grósz, St. von: Eponyme-syndrome. Klin. Monatsbl. Augenheilkd. *148*, 1–45 (1966)

Hager, H.: Discussion of: Jochmus, H.: Fundusblutungen und Hornhauttrübungen bei Frühgeborenen. Klin. Monatsbl. Augenheilkd. *152*, 106 (1968)

Harcourt, B., Hopkins, D.: Ophthalmic manifestations of the battered-baby syndrome. Br. Med. J. *3*, 398–401 (1971)

Harcourt, B., Hopkins, D.: Permanent chorio-retinal lesions in childhood of suspected traumatic origin. Trans. Ophthalmol. Soc. U.K. *93*, 199–205 (1973)

Hayreh, S.S.: Pathogenesis of oedema of the optic disc (papilloedema). Br. J. Ophthalmol. *48*, 522–543 (1964)

Heath, P.: Retrolental fibroplasia as a syndrome: Pathogenesis and classifications. A.M.A. Arch. Ophthalmol. *44*, 245–274 (1950)

Heath, P.: Pathology of the retinopathy of prematurity: Retrolental fibroplasia. Am. J. Ophthalmol. *34*, 1249–1259 (1951)

Hedges, T.R., Weinstein, J.D., Crystle, C.D.: Orbital vascular response to acutely increased intracranial pressure in the rhesus monkey. Arch. Ophtalmol. *71*, 226–237 (1964)

Hervouet, F.: Les hématomes sous-duraux du nourisson et leurs répercussions rétiniennes. Travaux d'anatomie pathologique oculaire. Paris: Masson 1968, pp. 68–82

Hickl, E.-J.: Comparative investigations into the significance of fibrinolysis inhibitors for the prevention of fetal hypoxic haemorrhages. Proc. VI. World Congr. Obstet. Gynaecol (New York), 1970, p. 276

Hickl, E.-J.: Intrakranielle Neugeborenenblutungen und geburtshilfliche Operationen. Dtsch. Med. Wochenschr. *97*, 736–739 (1972)

Hickl, E.-J., Barsewisch, B. von: Der Einfluß der protrahierten Geburt auf das Kind. Vortrag, Internationaler Kongreß „Das spastisch gelähmte Kind". Düsseldorf, Okt. 1969

Hickl, E.-J., Barsewisch, B. von, Dirschinger: Untersuchungen zur Frage der Wirksamkeit von Fibrinolysehemmern für die Prophylaxe fetaler Hypoxieblutungen. Dtsch. Med. Wochenschr. *95*, 616–618; 627 (1970)

Hickl, E.-J., Grässel, G., Kugler, J., Fröschl, J., Fendel, H.: Neurologische, ophthalmologische und radiologische Untersuchungen bei Neugeborenen nach Vakuumextraktion. 37. Tagung der Dtsch. Ges. Gynäkol. (Lübeck–Travemünde) 1968. Excerpt: Arch. Gynäkol. *207*, 42 (1969)

Hippel, E. von: Pathologisch-anatomische Befunde am Auge des Neugeborenen. Graefes Arch. Ophthalmol. *45*, 313–321 (1898)

Hogan, M.J., Alvarado, J.A., Weddell: Histology of the human eye. Philadelphia–London–Toronto: Saunders 1971

Hogan, M.J., Feeney, L.: Ultrastructure of the retinal blood vessels. J. Ultrastructure Res. *9*, 10–64 (1963)

Hogan, M.J., Zimmerman, L.E.: Ophthalmic pathology, an atlas and textbook, 2. ed. Philadelphia–London: Saunders 1962

Honegger, H.: Der Augenhintergrund bei Neu- und Frühgeborenen. Ber. Dtsch. Ophthalmol. Ges. *69*, 156–158 (1969)

Hoo, L.K.: Retinal haemorrhages in newborns after delivery with the vacuum-extractor. Trans. Ophthalmol. Soc. N.Z. *25*, 36–38 (1973)

Hosaka, A.: The ocular findings in the premature infants, especially on the premature signs. Jpn. J. Ophthalmol. *7*, 77–81 (1963)

Humblet, M., Cavrot, E., Richard, J.: L'hémorragie rétinienne du nouveau-né à terme. Bull. Soc. Belge Ophthalmol. *110*, 140–141 (1955)

Ishikawa, H.: About retinal hemorrhages in the newborn. Ganka Rinsho Iho *53*, 893–895 (1959)

Jacobs, M.W.: Retinal hemorrhage in the new-born. J. Am. Med. Assoc. *83*, 1641–1645 (1924)

Jacobs, M.W.: The frequency in the newborn of intraocular hemorrhages and their relationship to intracranial trauma. Trans. Am. Acad. Opthalmol. Otolaryngol, 33rd Annual Meeting, 218–226 (1928)

Jacobs, M.W.: Ocular birth injuries. N.Y. State J. Med. *30*, 1355–1358 (1930)

Jaeger, E. von: Über die Einstellungen des dioptrischen Apparates im menschlichen Auge. 2nd ed. Wien: Seidel 1861

Jaeger, E.: Ergebnisse der Untersuchungen mit dem Augenspiegel. Wien: L.W. Seidel, 1976

Jain, I.S., Gupta, A.N.: Retinal haemorrhages in the newborn. Proc. All. India Ophthalmol. Soc. *22*, 119–128 (1965)

Jain, I.S., Gupta, A.N.: Retinal haemorrhages in the newborn. Orient. A. Ophthalmol. *3*, 121–128 (1965)

Jarny, J.: Contribution à l'étude des hémorrhagies rétiniennes du nouveau-né. Paris: Thèse 1947, 64 p.

Jirman: Pediatr. Lysty (Praha) *117* (1947). Cited from: Lomickova, L., Otradovec, J.: Retinal hemorrhage in the newborn. CSL. Ofthalmol. *12*, 190–197 (1956)

Jochmus, H.: Fundusblutungen und Hornhauttrübungen bei Frühgeborenen. Manuscript, 5 p. Württ. Augenärztl. Vereinigung, 53. Tagung (Tübingen) 1967

Joppich, G., Schulte, F.J.: Neurologie des Neugeborenen. Berlin–Heidelberg–New York: Springer 1968

Juler, F.: Retinal haemorrhage in the newborn. Discussion on birth injuries of the eye, opening paper. Trans. Ophthalmol. Soc. U.K. *46*, 42–52 (1926)

Juler, F.: Discussion of: Richman, F.: Retinal haemorrhages in the newborn. Proc. R. Soc. Med. (London) *30*, 278–179 (1937)

Kästner, M.: Beobachtungen bei Frühgeburten. Klin. Monatsbl. Augenheilkd. *130*, 304–310 (1957)

Kauffman, M.L.: Observations on eyegrounds of the newborn. Pennsylv. Med. J., Sept. 1941, reprint, 5 p.

Kauffman, M.L.: Retinal hemorrhages in the newborn. Am. J. Ophthalmol. *46*, 658–660 (1958)

Kawakami, H., Oouchi, H., Yoshida, S., Takahashi, F., Inoguchi, T., Endo, M., Ono, K., Hara, K.: About retinal haemorrhage in the newborn. J. Jpn. Obstet. Gynecol. Soc. *15*, 801 (1963)

Kennedy, J.E., Wise, G.N.: Clinicopathological correlation of retinal lesions: Subacute bacterial endocarditis. Arch. Ophthalmol. *74*, 658–662 (1965)

Kerpel-Fronius, Ö.: Orv. Lapja (Budapest) *2*, 1253 (1946). cited from: Puskás, E., Szabó, Z.: Fundus-examinations of the newborn. Magy Nöorv. Lap. *6*, 334–343 (1961)

Khan, S.G., Frenkel, M.: Intravitreal hemorrhage associated with rapid increase in intracranial pressure (Terson's syndrome). Am. J. Ophthalmol. *80*, 37–43 (1975)

Ko, Ch.: Retinal haemorrhages in the newborn. Acta Soc. Ophthalmol. Jpn. *29*, 616 (1924); *30*, 117 (1925)

Kobayashi, T., Koomoto, H., Amano, K.: Examinations of retinal haemorrhages in the newborn. Obstet. Gynecol. *39*, 646–650 (1964)

Königstein, L.: Untersuchungen an den Augen neugeborener Kinder. Wiener Med. Jahrbücher, 47–70 (1881)

Konstantopais, K.G.: Retinal haemorrhages in the newborn. Athens: Dissertation 1956, 38 p.

Koyama, T.: Examination of retinal haemorrhages in the newborn. World Obstet. Gynecol. *11*, 883–892 (1959)

Kozcuhowska, J.: Retinal hemorrhages in the newborn. Post. Okul. (Kraków) *1*, 167 177 (1954)

Krauer-Mayer, B.: Retinahämorrhagien beim Neugeborenen. Gynaecologia (Basel) *160*, 61–65 (1965a)

Krauer-Mayer, B.: Retinahaemorrhagien beim Neugeborenen. Vergleichende Untersuchungen nach Spontangeburten, Vakuumextraktionen und Forceps. Ann. Paediatr. (Basel) *204*, 168–176 (1965b)

Krauer, F.: Über die Häufigkeit von Retinahämorrhagien beim Neugeborenen nach Forcepsentbindung und Vakuumextraktion. Gynaecologia (Basel) *160*, 56–60 (1965)

Krause, W., Krebs, W., Nestler, A., Thieme, G., Volkmer, H.: Untersuchungen über die Senkung der perinatalen Morbidität im Gefolge der kontinuierlichen elektronischen Geburtsüberwachung an Hand von Augenhintergrunduntersuchungen bei Kindern nach Risikogeburten in Gegenüberstellung zu sonstigen Geburten. Zentralbl. Gynäkol. *96*, 391–397 (1974)

Krebs, W., Jäger, G.: Netzhautblutungen bei Neugeborenen und Geburtsverlauf. Klin. Monatsbl. Augenheilkd. *148*, 483–490 (1966)

Krimsky, E.: Children's eye problems. New York–London: Grune and Straton 1956

Künzer, W.: Zur Physiologie der Blutgerinnung bei Neugeborenen. Dtsch. Med. Wochenschr. *89*, 1005–1010; 1077–1080 (1964)

Lachmann, G.S.: Bilateral hemorrhagic detachment of retina in the new born simulating glioma. Am. J. Ophthalmol. *10*, 164–167 (1927)

Lagrange, F., Valude, E. (eds.): Hémorrhagies rétiniennes par congestion passagère des vaisseaux. Encyclopédie française d'ophthalmologie, Vol. VI. Paris: Doin 1906, pp. 789–791

Larsen, H.W.: Discussion of: Nordentoft, V., Dalsgård, I.-L.: Retinal haemorrhages in the newborn. Acta Ophthalmol. (Kbh.) *47*, 270 (1969)

Laupus, W.E., Bousquet, F.P.: Retrolental fibroplasia; the role of hemorrhage in its pathogenesis. Am. J. Child. *81*, 617–626 (1951)

Leber, Th.: Die Krankheiten der Netzhaut. In: Handbuch der gesamten Augenheilkunde. Graefe, A., Saemisch, T. (eds.), 2nd ed., Vol. VII, Part II, Chap. X.A., 1st half, pp. 517–519. Leipzig: Engelmann 1915

Lemmingson, W., Stark, G.: Zur Klinik und Ätiologie der Netzhautblutungen bei Neugeborenen. Geburtshilfe Frauenheilkd. *17*, 548–557 (1957)

Lequeux: Examens ophthalmoscopiques chez le nouveau-né. Ann. Gynécol. Obstétr. (Paris) *8*, 740 (1911)

Lieb, W.A., Bielefeld, G.: Anatomie, Histologie und Physiologie der Endstromgefäße am Augenhintergrund. Med. Welt *18*, 742–748 (1967)

Liebrecht: Schädelbruch und Auge. Arch. Augenheilkd. *55*, 36–90 (1906)

Lomičková, H., Otradovec, J.: Retinal haemorrhage in the newborn. ČSL. Ofthalmol. *12*, 190–197 (1956)

Loriaux, C., Toussaint, D.: Hémorrhagies rétiniennes du nouveau-né et utilisation de la ventouse suédoise. Gynécol. Obstét. (Paris) *70*, 409–420 (1971)

Lowes, M., Ehlers, N., Jansen, I.K.: Visual functions after perinatal macular haemorrhage. Acta Ophthalmol. *54*, 227–232 (1976)

Lucas, W.P., Dearing, B.F., Hoobler, H.R., Cox, A., Jones, M.R., Smyth, F.S.: Blood studies in newborn: Morphology, chemical coagulation. Am. J. Dis. Child. *22*, 525–559 (1921)

Ludwig, H.: Mikrozirkulationsstörungen und Diapedeseblutungen im fetalen Gehirn bei Hypoxie. Fortschr. Geburtshilfe Gynäkol. *33*, 1–168 (1968)

Lukaszewicz, B.: Sequelae of retinal haemorrhages in 30 newborn. Klin. Oczna *42*, 1259–1261 (1972)

Lukaszewicz, B., Zaporowski, E.: Retinal haemorrhage in newborn. Klin. Oczna *39*, 43–49 (1969)

Luptakova, M.: Fundus oculi in new-born children. Čs. Oftalmol. *28*, 28–30 (1972)

McDonald, A.E.: Ocular lesions caused by intracranial hemorrhage. Trans. Am. Ophthalmol. Soc. *29*, 418–432 (1931)

Maertens, K., Götz, F.: Les hémorrhagies rétiniennes du nouveau-né africain. Gynaecologia (Basel) *167*, 71–82 (1967)

Manschot, W.A., Hampe, J.F.: The origin of ocular symptoms in spontaneous subarachnoid haemorrhages. XVI. Concilium Ophthalmologicum 1950, Britannia. Acta, Vol. 1, pp. 356–368 (1951)

Manschot, W.A.: Subarachnoid hemorrhage, intraocular symptoms and their pathogenesis. Am. J. Ophthalmol. *38*, 501–505 (1954)

Mao Wen-shu: Retinal hemorrhages in the newborn. Chin. J. Ophthalmol. *9*, 163–167 (1959). Excerpt: China Med. J. *78*, 394–395 (1959)

Martinez de Carbonnell, F., Grom, E.: Fondo ocular en los recién nacidos extraido por forceps. Arch. Soc. Oftalmol. Hisp. Amer. *29*, 917–924 (1969)

Martius, G.: Geburtsleitung bei gefährdeten Kindern. Münch. Med. Wochenschr. *107*, 657–662 (1965)

Martius, H.: Lehrbuch der Geburtshilfe. 7. ed. Stuttgart: G. Thieme 1971

Maumenee, A.E., Hellman, L.M., Shettles, L.B.: Factors influencing plasma prothrombin in the newborn infant. IV. The effect of antenatal administration of vitamin K on the incidence of retinal hemorrhage in the newborn. Johns Hopkins Med. J. *68*, 158–168 (1941)

Mayer, M., Maria, Y.: Les hémorrhagies rétiniennes du nouveau-né. Rapports XVème Congrès Féd. Soc. Gynécol. Obstét. Fr. (1952). Bull. Fed. Soc. Gynecol. Obstet. Fr. *4* (Suppl. 1), 259–265 (1952)

McKeown, H.S.: Retinal hemorrhages in the newborn. A.M.A. Arch. Ophthalmol. *26*, 25–37 (1941)

Metzger: Experimentelle Untersuchungen zur Genese der Netzhautblutungen der Neugeborenen. Dtsch. Med. Wochenschr. *51*, 1446–1447 (1925)

Mezey, P.: Szemeszet *89*, 39 (1952). Cited from: Puskás, E., Szabó, Z.: Fundus-examination of the newborn. Magy. Nöorv. Lap. *6*, 334–343 (1961)

Mijares, I.: Eye grounds in the new-borns. XVIII. Concil. Ophthalmol. Belgica 1958. Acta *2*, 1322–1324 (1959)

Millán, A.M., Beltrán San Martín, S.: Las hemorragias retinales en el recién nacido. Rev. Chilena Pediatr. *21*, 209–218 (1950)

Miller, A.J., Cuttino, J.T.: On the mechanism of production of massive preretinal hemorrhage following rupture of a congenital medial-defect intra-cranial aneurysm. Am. J. Ophthalmol. *31*, 15–24 (1948)

Minckler, D.S., Tso, M.O.M.: Experimental papilledema produced by cyclocryotherapy. Am. J. Ophthalmol. *82*, 577–589 (1976)

Minkowski, A.: Essai de prévention des hémorrhagies cérébro-méningées des prématurés par l'administration à la mère, pendant le travail, de substances "anti-fragilité vasculaire". Arch. Fr. Pédiatr. *6*, 276–280 (1949)

Montalcini: Di una interessante lesione in occhi dei neonati de della sua eziologia studiata spezialmente sotto il punto di ostetrica. Riv. Ostetr. (1897). Cited from: Jahresber. f. Augenheilk. *28*, 262 (1897)

Motohashi, T., Kobayashi, A.: About retinal haemorrhage in the newborn. Jpn. J. Clin. Ophthalmol. *14*, 775–783 (1960)

Moulène, C.: Contribution à l'étude des hémorrhagies rétiniennes du nouveau-né. Bordeaux: Thèse 1965, 39 pp.

Murillo Fajardo, R., Murillo, M.L.: Secuelas oftalmoscopicas en aplicación de forceps y cesáreas, observaciones en 450 recién nacidos. Arch. As. Evit. Ceguera Mexico *10*, 105–130 (1968)

Müschenhorn, I.: Zur Frage der Hirnblutungen bei Frühgeborenen. München: Dissertation 1970, 36 pp.

Nakajima, Y.: About retinal haemorrhages in the newborn. Sogoganka *38*, 60–65 (1943)

Nakayama, K.: Ophthalmological observations of premature infants. Folia Ophthalmol. Jpn. *14*, 546–555 (1963)

Naumoff, M.: Über einige pathologisch-anatomische Veränderungen im Augengrunde bei neugeborenen Kindern. Arch. Ophthalmol. *36*, 180–246 (1890)

Naunton, W.J., Forrester, R.M.: Severe vitreous haemorrhage in a premature infant. Br. J. Ophthalmol. *39*, 563–565 (1955)

Nehrdich, G.: Discussion of: Buchhalter, I., Schnecke, D.: Beitrag zur Problematik der Fundusblutungen bei Neugeborenen. Sitzung der Berliner Augenärztl. Ges., Dezember 1967. Klin. Monatsbl. Augenheilkd. *153*, 133 (1968)

Neme, B., Fraga, E., Salomao, A.J., Atzingen, I.V., Doneto Santos, E.P.: Efeitos da assistencia ao parto sôbre o sistema vascular fetal (5 consecutive chapters). Maternidade Infancia *31*, 5–24 (1972)

Neuweiler, N., Onwudiwe, E.U.: Retinahämorrhagien beim Neugeborenen. Gynaecologica (Basel) *163*, 27–42 (1967)

Nevinny-Stickel, H.: Über Geburtstraumen. Geburtshilfe Frauenheilkd. *14*, 1035–1041 (1954)

Niedermeier, S.: Experimentelle Untersuchungen zur Pathogenese der Stauungspapille. Graefes Arch. Ophthalmol. *157*, 397–406 (1956)

Nobiling, A.: Der pathologisch-anatomische Befund bei dem Erstickungstode des Neugeborenen und seine Verwerthung in gerichtlich-medicinischer Beziehung. Ärztliches Intelligenzblatt, Münch. Med. Wochenschr. *31*, 417–421; 431–432; 442–446 (1884)

Noorden, G.K. von, Khohadoust, A.: Retinal haemorrhage in newborns and organic amblyopia. Arch. Ophthalmol. *89*, 91–93 (1973)

Noorden, G.K. von, Maumenee, E.: Atlas der Schieldiagnostik. Translated by Noorden, G.K. von. Stuttgart-New York: Schattauer 1971

Nordentoft, V., Dalsgård, I.-L.: Retinal haemorrhages in the newborn. Acta Ophthalmol. (Kbh.) *47*, 269–270 (1969)

Oliver, M., Nawratzki, I.: Screening of pre-school children for ocular anomalies, II. Amblyopia. Prevalence and therapeutic results at different ages. Br. J. Ophthalmol. *55*, 467–471 (1971)

Orduña, G., De Arizcun Pineda, J.: El fondo de ojo como indice de valoración de las diferentes técnicas de parto. Arch. Soc. Oftalmol. Hisp. Amer. *30*, 271–276 (1970)

Pajor, R., Szabó, Z., Puskás, E.: Control examination at 3 years of age in 227 infants with retinal hemorrhages at birth. Orv. Hetil. Budapest *105*, 781–783 (1964)

Panagiotou, P.P., Georgiadi, G., Kologeropoulo, A., Tsigdinou, X.: Fundus haemorrhages in the eyes of newborn infants after natural delivery and after cesarian section. Arch. Ophthalmol. Soc. (Northern Greece) *17*, 181–200 (1968)

Pannarale, P.: Rilievi clinico-statistici sulle emorragie retiniche nel neonato. Minerva Oftalmol. *8*, 1–8 (1966)

Papoušek: Conference Cechoslovak Gynecol. Soc., February 1954. Cited from: Lomičková, H., Otradovec, I.: Retinal haemorrhage in the newborn. CSL. Ofthalmol. *12*, 190–197 (1956)

Paufique, L., Ravault, M.-P., Bonnet, M., Picaud, M.H.: Les hémorrhagies rétiniennes des nouveau-né: Essai d'interprétation physio-pathogénique. Bull. Soc. Ophthalmol. Fr. *65*, 150–155 (1965)

Paul, A.: Über einige Augenspiegelbefunde bei Neugeborenen. Halle: Inaugural-Dissertation 1900, 20 pp.

Paunoff: Glaskörperblutung bei Subarachnoidalblutung (Terson-Syndrom). Klin. Monatsbl. Augenheilkd. *141*, 625 (1962)

Péhu, Bonamour, G.: Sur les hémorrhagies rétiniennes observees chez le nouveau-né. Bull. Acad. Méd. (Paris) *120*, 760–764 (1938)

Pentini, G.: Atti XXI. Congr. Ital. Pediat., Venezia, 15–19 sept. 1951. Cited from: Dorello, U., Poli, L.: L'aspetto oftalmoscopico del fundus nel neonato prematuro. Arch. Oftalmol. *17*, 17–23 (1953)

Peters, A.: Eine Verletzung der Hornhaut durch Zangenentbindung mit anatomischem Befund. Arch. Augenheilkd. *56*, 311–319 (1907)

Phelps, C.D.: The association of pale-centered retinal hemorrhages with intracranial bleeding in infancy. Am. J. Ophthalmol. *72*, 348–350 (1971)

Pietrowa, N.: Haemorrhages of the retina in newborn babies. Klin. Oczna *26*, 67–82 (1956). Excerpt: Ophthalmol. Lit. *10*, 72 (1956)

Planten, J.Th., Schaaf, P.C. v.d.: Retinal hemorrhage in the newborn. An attempt to indicate and explain its cause and significance. Ophthalmologica (Basel) *162*, 213–222 (1971)

Podestà, H.H., Ullerich, K.: Demonstration zur Gefäßanatomie der Netzhaut. Ber. Dtsch. Ophthalmol. Ges. *60*, 270–272 (1956)

Pöllmann, A.: Augenhintergrund und Funktion nach perinatalen Maculablutungen. München: Dissertation 1979 (in preparation)

Pommer, H.: Die Geburt als Ursache von kindlichen Netzhautblutungen. Klin. Monatsbl. Augenheilkd. *160*, 203–206 (1972)

Pontorieri, N., Conciliis, U. de: Rilievi clinico-statistici sullo piccole emorragie, con particolare riguardo alle emorragie retiniche nel neonato. Lattante *30*, 257–309 (1959)

Powelett, A.C., Townes, C.D.: Intra-ocular hemorrhage in the newborn. Kentucky Med. J. *46*, 420–423 (1948)

Pray, L.G., McKeown., H.S., Pollard, W.E.: Hemorrhagic diathesis of the newborn. Am. J. Obstet. Gynecol. *42*, 836–845 (1941)

Puskás, E., Szabó, Z.: Fundus-examinations of the newborn. Magy. Nöorv. Lap. *6* (?), 334–343 (1961)

Pushkash, E., Sabo, Z.: Examination of the fundus in the newborn. Akušerstvo Ginekol. *5* (?), 76–79 (1962)

Reese, A.B., Blodi, F.C., Locke, J.C.: The pathology of early retrolental fibroplasia with an analysis of the histologic findings in the eyes of newborn and stillborn infants. Am. J. Ophthalmol. *35*, 1407–1426 (1952)

Remky, H.: Discussion of: Barsewisch, B. von, Hickl, E.-J.: Retinalblutungen bei Neugeborenen. Klin. Monatsbl. Augenheilkd. *159*, 121 (1971)

Remky, H., Schum, U.: Fluoreszenz-Angiographie am liegenden Patienten. Klin. Monatsbl. Augenheilkd. *153*, 589–591 (1968)

Richman, F.: Retinal haemorrhages in the newborn. Proc. R. Soc. Med. *30*, 277–280 (1937a)

Richman, F.: Ophthalmoscopic study of newborn infants' eyes. XV. Conc. Ophthalmol. 1937, Egypte, T. IV, pp. 76–86

Richter, S.: Über die Bedeutung ophthalmologischer Untersuchungen bei Neugeborenen. Wissenschaftl. Z. Univ. Rostock *18*, M 9/10, part 1, 1061–1063 (1969)

Rico, M.: Sur les hémorrhagies rétiniennes du nouveau-né. Lyon: Thèse 1939, 72 pp.

Riddoch, G., Goulden, C.: On the relationship between subarachnoid and intraocular haemorrhage. Br. J. Ophthalmol. *9*, 209–233 (1925)

Rohen, J.W.: Morphologie. In: Der Augenarzt. Velhaken, K. (ed.), 2nd ed., Vol. I. Leipzig: G. Thieme 1969

Rowland, W.D.: Ocular pathology of the newborn. Am. J. Ophthalmol. *10*, 824–828 (1927)

Rowland, W.D.: Ocular pathology of the newborn, and end-results study. Am. J. Ophthalmol. *18*, 647–650 (1935)

Runge, E.: Gynäkologie und Geburtshilfe in ihren Beziehungen zur Ophthalmologie. Leipzig: J.A. Barth 1908

Rupprecht, J.: Über multiple isolierte Risse der Descemet'schen Membran als Geburtsverletzung. Klin. Monatsbl. Augenheilkd. *46*, 134–139 (1908)

Sachsenweger, R.: Über die Ursachen der Schielamblyopie. Klin. Monatsbl. Augenheilkd. *147*, 499–489 (1965)

Sachsenweger, R.: Untersuchung über die Störungen im retinalen Blutkreislauf bei Neugeborenen. In: Proc. XX Int. Congr. Ophthalmol., Munich 1966. Weigelin, E. (ed.). Amsterdam: Excerpta Med. Found. 1967, pp. 268–269

Sachsenweger, R.: Round table session I. In: International Strabismus Symposium. Arruga, A. (ed.). Basel–New York: Karger 1968, p. 78

Sanchez-Ibanez, J.M., Belmonte Gonzales, N., Navarro Martinez, A.: Retina-Hämorrhagien beim Neugeborenen nach Vakuum-Extraktion. Gynaecologia (Basel) *156*, 172–186 (1963)

Sanford, H.N.: The effect of gas anesthetics used in labor. J. Am. Med. Assoc. *86*, 265–267 (1926)

Sanford, H.H., Shmigelsky, I., Chapin, J.M.: Is administration of vitamin K to the newborn of clinical value? J. Am. Med. Assoc. *118*, 697–702 (1942)

Santamarina, J.M.: Hemorragias retinianas del recién nacido. Relación con los factores obstétricos. Arch. Soc. Oftalmol. Hisp. Amer. *29*, 421–430 (1969)

Sasaki, T.: Studies on amblyopia. Relation of retinal hemorrhage in new born and occurrence of amblyopia. Jpn. J. Clin. Ophthalmol. *25*, 819–825 (1971)

Schenk, H., Stangler-Zuschrott, E.: Die Auswirkungen zentraler Netzhautblutungen beim Neugeborenen auf Sehvermögen und Muskelgleichgewicht. Klin. Monatsbl. Augenheilkd. *165*, 867–870 (1974)

Schenker, J.G., Gombos, G.M.: Retinal hemorrhage in the newborn. Obstet. Gynecol. *27*, 521–524 (1966)

Schlaeder, G., Gerhard, J.P., Mot, M. de, Payeur, G., Gandar, R.: Les hémorrhagies rétiniennes chez le nouveau-né après accouchement par ventouse et accouchement spontané. Gynécol. Obstét. (Paris) *70*, 95–108 (1971)

Schleich: Die Augen hundertfünfzig neugeborener Kinder ophthalmoskopisch untersucht. Mittheilungen aus der ophthalmiatrischen Klinik in Tübingen *2*, 44–56 (1884)

Schmidt, B., Trojan, H.J.: Augenhintergrundsbefunde und histologische Untersuchungen bei der Pachymeningosis haemorrhagica interna des Kindes. Klin. Monatsbl. Augenheilkd. *157*, 239–244 (1970)

Schwartz, Ph.: Birth injuries of the newborn. Basel–New York: S. Karger 1961

Seefelder: Discussion of: Sicherer, von: Ophthalmoskopische Untersuchungen Neugeborener. Ber. Dtsch. Ophthalmol. Ges. *34*, 216 (1907)

Seissiger, J.: Augenbefunde bei Neugeborenen. Arch. Augenheilkd. *100*, 302–313 (1929)

Seitz, R.: Klinik und Pathologie der Netzhautgefäße. Stuttgart: F. Enke 1968

Sezen, F.: Retinal haemorrhages in newborn infants. Br. J. Ophthalmol. *55*, 248–253 (1970)

Sicherer, von: Ophthalmoskopische Untersuchungen Neugeborener. Ber. Dtsch. Ophthalmol. Ges. *34*, 201–218 (1907)

Sidler-Huguenin: Beitrag zur Kenntnis der Geburtsverletzungen des Auges. Correspondenzbl. f. Schweiz. Aerzte *33*, 169–175; 205–213 (1903)

Singer, G., Sgallová, I., Kudrnovský, J.: Retinal haemorrhages in the newborn. Čsl. Ofthalmol. *12*, 184–189 (1956)

Smith, D.C., Kearns, T.P., Sayre, G.P.: Preretinal and optic nerve-sheath haemorrhage: Pathologic and experimental aspects in subarachnoid haemorrhage. Trans. Am. Acad. Ophthalmol. Otolaryngol. *61*, 201–211 (1957)

Sopanen, V.: On retinal haemorrhages in newborns. Acta Ophthalmol. (Kbh.) *44*, 702 (1966)

Sorsby, A. (ed.): Modern ophthalmology, Vol. II, p. 595. London: Butterworths 1963

Sourdille, J.: Le fond d'oeil dans les hématomes sous-duraux du nourrisson. Bull. Soc. Ophthalmol. Fr. *64*, 158–170 (1964)

Sourdille, J.: Discussion of Fritz, A., Parent, G., Lambiliotte, A., Beckmann, G.: Physiopathologie des hémorrhagies rétiniennes obstétricales. Bull. Coc. Belge Ophthalmol. *142*, 487–489 (1966)

Stefanini, U., Ferruti, M., Rankel, G., Ricci, P.: Contributo allo studio delle emorragie retiniche nel neonato. Minverva Nipiol. *18*, 110–112 (1968)

Štefek, J.: Reinal haemorrhages in the newborn. Čsl. Gynaekol. *16*, 156–158 (1951)

Štefek, J.: Prognostic evaluation of retinal haemorrhages in the newborn. Acta Univ. Palackianae Olomucensis *10*, 187–194 (1956)

Stocker, F.: Über ophthalmoskopische Betrachtungen an durch Sectio caesarea geborenen Kindern. Schweiz. Med. Wochenschr. *57*, 1096–1099 (1927)

Stumpf, M., Sicherer, von: Über Blutungen ins Auge bei Neugeborenen. Beitr. Geburtshilfe Gynäkol. *13*, 408–429 (1909)

Sykes, C.S.: A study of retinal findings in the new born. Tex. J. Med. *26*, 878–883 (1931)

Symonds, C.P.: Spontaneous subarachnoid hemorrhage. Q. J. Med. *18*, 93 (1924). Cited from: Miller, A.J., Cuttino, J.T.: On the mechanism of production of massive preretinal hemorrhage following rupture of a con-genital medial-defect intra-cranial aneurysm. Am. J. Ophthalmol. *31*, 15–24 (1948)

Szewczyk, T.S.: Retrolental fibroplasia and related ocular diseases. Am. J. Ophthalmol. *36*, 1336–1361 (1953)

Szirmák, E., Rajk, A., Pajor, R.: Fundusuntersuchungen bei Frühgeburten und reifen Neugeborenen. Med. Monatsschr. *25*, 216–219 (1971)

Tadashi, K., Fujimori, H.: About fundus observations in the newborn. Sanfujinka Kiyo (Gynäkologische Zeitschrift) *22*, 1462 (1941)

Takala, M.E., Sopanen, V.: Retinal haemorrhages in the newborn. Duodecim *83*, 1413–1418 (1967)

Takeda, K.: Retinal haemorrhages in the newborn of painless delivery by inhalation anesthesia. Jpn. J. Clin. Ophthalmol. *22*, 217–230 (1968)

Taleb Bendiab, M.A.: Contribution à l'étude des hémorrhagies rétiniennes du nouveauné. Alger: Thèse 1972, 54 pp.

Tanaka, S.: Untersuchungen über die gynäkologische und klinische Anwendung des EEG bei Neugeborenen. Brain Nerve *18*, 1016–1069 (1966)

Terado, H.: About the influence of vitamin K on retinal haemorrhages of the newborn. J. Jpn. Obstet. Gynecol. *5*, 883–889 (1953)

Terson, A.: Le syndrome de l'hématome du corps vitré et de l'hémorrhagie intracranienne spontanée. Ann. Oculist. *163*, 666–673 (1926)

Thomson, W.E., Buchanan, L.: A clinical and pathological account of some of the injuries to the eye of the child during labour. Trans. Ophthalmol. Soc. U.K. *23*, 296–319 (1903)

Toussaint, D., Kuwabara, T., Cogan, D.: Retinal vascular patterns. A.M.A. Arch. Ophthalmol. *65*, 575–581 (1961)

Tranou-Sphalangakou, L.: About retinal haemorrhages in the newborn. Athens: Habilitation-Thesis 1968, 84 pp.

Treit, S., Stefanics, D., Csömor, S., Dömötöri, J.: Fundus examinations of newborn infants with special regard of vacuum extractions. Magyar Nöorvosok Lapja *27*, 142–145 (1964)

Truc, H.: Lésions obstétricales de l'oeil et de ses annexes. Ann. Oculist (Paris) *119*, 161–174 (1898)

Tsópelas, B., Charamis, H.: Hemorrhages of the retina in newborn children. Bull. Soc. Hellen. Ophthalmol. *23*, 173–185 (1955)

Tyner, G.S.: Ophthalmoscopic findings in normal premature infants. Arch. Ophthalmol. *45*, 627–629 (1952)

Ulrich, G.: Refraction und Papilla optica der Augen der Neugeborenen. Königsberg: Inaugural-Dissertation 1884

Unger, L.: Begleitschielen und frühkindlicher Hirnschaden. Klin. Monatsbl. Augenheilkd. *130*, 642–659 (1957)

Vancea, P.: Die Netzhautblutungen des Neugeborenen. Klin. Monatsbl. Augenheilkd. *107*, 272–274 (1941)

Vancea, P.: Discussion of: Sachsenweger, R.: Untersuchungen über die Störungen im retinalen Blutkreislauf bei Neugeborenen. Proc. XX Int. Congr. Ophthalmol., München, 1966. Weigelin, E. (ed.). Amsterdam: Excerpta Med. Found. 1967, p. 269

Veinbaum, D.S.: Treatment of haemorrhages of the fundus of newborn babies. Oftalmol. Zh. *22*, 579–582 (1967)

Velhagen, K. (ed.): Der Augenarzt, Vol. VI, p. 234. Leipzig: G. Thieme 1964

Vincenti, F., Gavinelli, R.: Il fondo dell'occhio del neonato. Minerva Ginecol. *21*, 426–427 (1969a)

Vincenti, F., Gavinelli, R.: L'esame del fondo dell'occhio del neonato. Minerva Ginecol. *21*, 608–613 (1969b)

Voegeli, H.: Pratique de L'extraction par ventouse à la maternité de Genève. Gynéc. Obstét. *57*, 95–104 (1958)

Ward, B.A.: Ocular histology in premature infants with reference to retrolental fibroplasia. Br. J. Ophthalmol. *38*, 445–459 (1954)

Walsh, F.B., Fletcher Hoyt, W.: Clinical neuro-ophthalmology, 3rd ed., Vol. III, pp. 2340–2341. Baltimore: Williams and Wilkins 1969

Wecker, L. de: Les lésions oculaires obstétricales. Ann. Ocul. (Paris) *116*, 40–45 (1896)

Wehrli, E.: Über die Beziehungen der während der Geburt entstehenden Retinablutungen des Kindes zur Pathogenese des Glioma retinae. Correspondenzbl. Schweiz. Ärzte *35*, 43–47 (1905)

Weiden, H.: Über Netzhautblutungen bei Neugeborenen mit unterschiedlichem Geburtsverlauf. Klin. Monatsbl. Augenheilkd. *156*, 363–371 (1970)

Wierhake, E.-S.: Über die Häufigkeit der retinalen und subconjunktivalen Blutungen bei Neugeborenen an der Universitäts-Frauenklinik Tübingen. Tübingen: Inaugural-Dissertation 1971, 63 + V pp.

Wille, H.: Investigations in the influence of K avitaminosis on the occurrence of retinal hemorrhages in the newborn. Acta Ophthalmol. *22*, 261–269 (1946)

Wintersteiner, H.: Beitrag zur Kenntnis der Geburtsverletzungen des Auges. Z. Augen-
heilkd. *2*, 443–454 (1899)
Wise, G.N., Dollery, C.T., Henkind, P.: The retinal circulation. New York: Harper and
Row 1971, 566 pp.
Wiznia, R.A., Price, J.: Vitreous hemorrhages and disseminated intravascular coagula-
tion in the newborn. Am. J. Ophthalmol. *82*, 222–226 (1976)
Wolff, B.: Injuries of the eyes of the child during labour. Ophthalmoscope *5*, 484–492;
584–588; 650–654; 712–718 (1907); *6*, 23–32; 88–96 (1908)
Wolff, E., Davies, F.: A contribution to the pathology of papilledema. Br. J. Ophthal-
mol. *15*, 609–632 (1931)
Yamanouchi, U.: About retinal haemorrhages in the newborn. Jpn. Monatsschr. prakt.
Augenheilk. *53*, 999–1002 (1959)
Yohitda, M., Yasuoka, T., Yoshida, S.: Statistic investigations on retinal haemorrhage
of new borns. Acta Soc. Ophthalmol. Jpn. *65*, 2411–2415 (1961)
Yoshioka, H.: Studies on the eyes of premature infants. I. On the histologic findings
of the eyes and autopsy findings. Acta Soc. Ophthalmol. Jpn. *58*, 879–904 (1954)
Zehetbauer, G.: Zur Zeitdauer der Entwicklung einer Stauungspapille bei Hirndruck-
steigerung. Klin. Monatsbl. Augenheilkd. *171*, 613 (1977)
Zgorzalewicz, T.: Haemorrhages into the retina of the newborn. Pol. Tyk. Lek. *29*,
2047–2048 (1974)
Zgorzalewicz, T., Kikiela, M., Poprawa, A.: Intraretinal hemorrhages in the newborn
delivered by natural forces and by vacuum extraction. Ginekol. Polska *46*, 641–
647 (1975)
Zisa, F., Capozzi, A., Ceccarello, P.L.: Incidenza delle lesioni vascolari retiniche con-
seguenti al parto. Minerva Ginecol. *27*, 294–297 (1975)

Subject Index

S.N. Hassani

Real Time Ophthalmic Ultrasonography

1978. Approx. 425 figures. Approx. 400 pages
Cloth DM 69,–; US $ 34.50
ISBN 3-540-90318-6

Contents: Principles of Ultrasonography. – Ophthalmic Anatomy. – Sonoanatomy. – Ultrasonic Patient History. – Oculosonotomography. – Sonography of the Injured Eye. – Sonography of the Lens. – Sonography of the Vitreous. – Sonography of the Retina and Choroid. – Sonography of the Optic Nerve. – Sonography of the Orbit. – Sonography of the Ophthalmic Tumors. – Sonography of the Eye in Systemic Disease. – Artifacts. – Glossary.

Here is a comprehensive survey of the principles of ultrasound physics and the practical aspects of scanning procedures in the eye and orbit. A new identification system optimizes localization of lesions in these two areas, simplifying three-dimensional depiction of ophthalmic pathology.

Methods of examination and the analysis of diagnostic findings are precisely explained with the ophthalmologist and radiologist in mind. A chapter devoted to ophthalmic ultrasonic anatomy highlights normal variants often mistaken for pathologic entities. And a section on ocular manifestations of systemic disorders is only one feature of this book which makes it an authoritative reference for the practicing clinician. *Real Time Ophthalmic Ultrasonography* serves as a link between sonographic imaging and ophthalmic pathology.

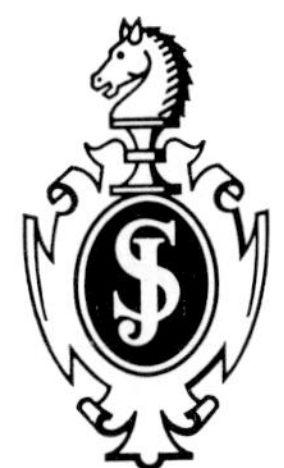

Springer-Verlag
Berlin
Heidelberg
New York

Topics in
Environmental
Physiology
and Medicine

Editor: K.E. Schaefer

F. Hollwich

The Influence of Ocular Light Perception on Metabolism in Man and in Animals

Translated from the German by H.G. Hannun,
H.K. Hannun
1978. Approx. 70 figures. Approx. 140 pages
Cloth DM 82,–; US $ 41.00
ISBN 3-540-90315-1

Contents: The "Energetic Portion" of the Optic Nerve. –
Light and the Pineal Organ. – Light and Color Change. –
Light and Growth. – Light and Body Temperature. – Light
and Kidney Function. – Light and Blood Count. – Light
and Metabolic Functions. – Light and Thyroid Function. –
Light and Sexual Function. – Light and Adrenal Func-
tion. – Light and Pituitary Hormones. – Natural Sunlight
and Artificial-Fluorescent Light. – Light Pollution. – The
Importance of Light in Metabolism in Man and Animals:
Summary.

It is today indisputable that both the absence of ocular
light perception (for example, in the blind) and overly intense illumination, such as artificial light, cause vegetative
and psychological disturbances. Light perceived by the eye
not only evokes optical impulses (appreciation of form and
color of the environment), but also has a second "energetic"
function which directly influences life processes.

This book investigates the influence of light perceived by
the eye on subconcious life processes governed by the vegetative nervous system. Areas under study were the effects of
the constant absence of light perception in blind persons
and its temporary absence in patients before and after
cataract operations, and the influence of daylight and artificial light on man and animals. Results show that natural
light has a stimulating effect on life processes. This effect
is, however, absend in blind people. Artificial light of the
strength of 1000 Lux has, on the other hand, a stress-like
effect on certain blood cells (eosinophils, thrombocytes).
Ocular light perception also influences water, protein, fat
and sugar metabolism, blood formation and blood count,
the function of the thyroid gland and of the adrenal glands,
as well as the sexual cycle and its secondary features.

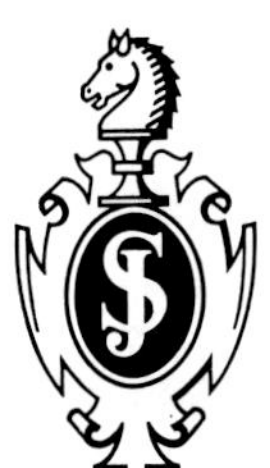

Springer-Verlag
Berlin
Heidelberg
New York